TIFFANY FLATTEN, CNS, LN

**The 8-Week
Thyroid Diet for
People with
"Normal" Thyroid
Test Results
to Thrive,
Not Just Survive**

Rock Bottom

THYROID

TREATMENT

Rock Bottom Wellness
www.rockbottomwellness.com

Publisher's Cataloging-In-Publication Data
(Prepared by The Donohue Group, Inc.)

Names: Flaten, Tiffany, author.
Title: Rock bottom thyroid treatment : an 8-week thyroid diet for people
    with "normal" thyroid test results to thrive, not just survive /
    Tiffany Flaten.
Description: [St Michael, Minnesota] : Rock Bottom Wellness, [2020] |
    Includes bibliographical references.
Identifiers: ISBN 9781734754308 (paperback) | ISBN 9781734754315
    (hardback) | ISBN 9781734754322 (ebook)
Subjects: LCSH: Thyroid gland--Diseases--Diet therapy. | Thyroid hormones.
    | Thyroid gland function tests. | Flaten, Tiffany--Health.
Classification: LCC RC655 .F53 2020 (print) | LCC RC655 (ebook) | DDC
    616.4/40654--dc23

Disclaimer

This book details the author's personal experiences with and opinions about physical and/or mental health. The author is not a healthcare provider. The author is providing this book and its contents on an "as is" basis and makes no representations or warranties of any kind with respect to this book or its contents. The author disclaims all such representations and warranties, including for example warranties of merchantability and healthcare for a particular purpose. In addition, the author does not represent or warrant that the information accessible via this book is accurate, complete, or current.

The statements made about products and services have not been evaluated by the US Food and Drug Administration (FDA). They are not intended to diagnose, treat, cure, or prevent any condition or disease. Please consult with your own physician or healthcare specialist regarding the suggestions and recommendations made in this book.

The author will not be liable for damages arising out of or in connection with the use of this book. This is a comprehensive limitation of liability that applies to all damages of any kind, including (without limitation) compensatory; direct, indirect, or consequential damages; loss of data, income, or profit; loss of or damage to property; and claims of third parties.

You understand that this book is not intended as a substitute for consultation with a licensed healthcare practitioner, such as your physician. Before you begin any healthcare program or change your lifestyle in any way, you will consult your physician or another licensed healthcare practitioner to ensure that you are in good health and that the examples contained in this book will not harm you.

This book provides content related to physical and/or mental health issues. As such, use of this book implies your acceptance of this disclaimer.

I dedicate this book to my husband and kids who supported and loved me through the hard times. I love you all.

Keep on Thriving

Your healing journey goes beyond the book.

If you're ready to get the personalized help you need to achieve sustainable health, reach out to me and let's schedule your free thirty-minute **Thyroid Breakthrough Session today**. Go to www.rockbottomwellness.com/breakthrough.

And if you want to join a community that feels like family, join my free group **Nutrition for Thyroid Health**. Just go to www.rockbottomwellness.com/group. Introduce yourself and ask the question that stumped your doctor.

Contents

Foreword

Did you know that women are five to eight times more likely than men to have thyroid problems? And that one in eight women develops a thyroid disorder during her lifetime?[1]

A chronic health issue may feel like the end of the world, but I can tell you from over two decades in traditional health promotion and comprehensive holistic wellness that your journey to an optimally healthy life has only begun.

That's where Tiffany Flaten comes in; I highly recommend her to anyone with a thyroid issue. Ever since we met in Mindshare and I interviewed her on Her Brilliant Health Radio, I've known Tiffany to be a wise, insightful, caring clinician who can help anyone get their health on track.

As a community OBGYN, I saw firsthand the overlap of hormonal health and thyroid health. In order for a woman to thrive in life, an elaborate hormonal balance must occur. One of those hormones is, of course, thyroid hormone. Weight gain, fatigue, constipation, thinning hair, and foggy thinking are just a few of the symptoms that can result when thyroid hormone levels are not optimized. Maybe your doctor has been checking minimal labs to follow you, meanwhile neglecting vital tests that could mean the difference between you surviving and

---

[1] "General Information/Press Room." American Thyroid Association. www.thyroid.org/media-main/press-room/.

actually thriving. Your labs say you're "normal," but you feel anything but that!

If you have a health problem, then you have a fuel problem because you don't have the energy to fix the problems that the body naturally wants to fix. Addressing key nutrient deficiencies is essential to having optimized thyroid function, health, and vitality. I am so excited about Rock Bottom Thyroid Treatment because Tiffany shares how she unlocked flourishing health through the right diet—and how you can, too.

Tiffany will walk you by the hand as you learn the nature of thyroid illness, how food sensitivities contribute to thyroid dysfunction, why gluten and wheat are particularly troublesome for thyroid disorders, which vital tests identify specific nutrient deficiencies, and much, much more.

You don't have to be reactive on your health journey. You can make positive change happen yourself, rise from rock bottom, and lead a life of wellness.

Kyrin Dunston MD FACOG

Host, Her Brilliant Health Revolution

Author, *Cracking the Bikini Code: 6 Secrets to Permanent Weight Loss Success*

R

CHAPTER 1

Thriving after a Diagnosis

"I just can't thank you enough for the info you sent, the time you spend listening to me, and the genuine concern you have for my health. I truly believe I have found my last Natural Care Practitioner. Can't wait to begin the journey, I promise to keep you updated."

— Luna K., Sante Fe, New Mexico

My Numbers Were Normal

I know what it's like to be sick.

For ten years, I felt depressed, frustrated, and hopeless. My days were clouded with general pissed-offness. I was wired yet somehow always exhausted. Not just tired. It was pregnancy fatigue every day. Mothers who remember their first trimester know what I'm talking about. My body felt weak. Like I was running a marathon every moment of every day.

Just moving the laundry from the washer to the dryer was a monumental task. Then I had to fold it. I would carry the basket to the couch thinking, *I'll fold while I watch TV.* Then I'd lie down and take a nap. I'd sit up an hour later, and pure adrenaline got me through folding. Then I'd have to take it up to the bedrooms and put it away. I could only do laundry on the weekends because it took me *all day* to finish this simple task.

I didn't want to do anything. I didn't want to socialize. I didn't want to exercise. I didn't want to go to work. I didn't even want to play with my kids. I felt anxious at work because I didn't want to be there. Then anxious coming home because I had to be "on" for my kids. Every day I couldn't wait to crawl into bed and do nothing. I felt like a house with all the curtains closed. Dark. Heavy.

What the hell happened to me? I'd always thought of myself as healthy. As a kid, I was fit, active, and normal. When high school happened, things changed. I got sick a lot. I never had the energy my friends did. Somehow I managed, and I went to college. Then my focus and mood tanked. I complained to my family doctor about always feeling miserable.

"You're busy," she said. "You're stressed. You're a college student. Anxiety is normal in your situation. Try to relax. That should help calm your anxiety."

Years passed. My struggles worsened. Depression, allergies, and chronic sinusitis tagged along with my anxiety. Then came the migraines. Terrible migraines.

My doctor referred me to a neurologist, who told me the cause was probably hormonal.

"A lot of women get migraines," he said.

"I don't know. They don't come on during my period," I said. "I haven't felt right for a while. I'm worried something else could be wrong . . ." I trailed off.

The neurologist smiled. "Don't worry so much. It's not that big of a deal. You're getting older. This stuff happens." He scribbled on a prescription pad. "Here's a medication that should take care of it."

I'm a college junior, and I'm "getting older"? Wow, I'm twenty, and I've already peaked. The diagnosis didn't make any sense. I was still at a healthy weight, and I exercised. I took the migraine medication, but it didn't help.

Around the time I graduated college and got married, I made an appointment with my family doctor to run lab tests. All my numbers came back normal, including my thyroid. Apparently, I was in perfect health. How frustrating is that?! You know how you *should* feel, and you see everyone around you living normal lives. For me, everything "normal" was a struggle.

I pushed my family doctor for a referral to a specialist, who diagnosed me with depression. Finally, a medication worked. I started to feel better. Not completely better, but the days felt easier. I took this small token of hope and tried to be proactive. I did whatever therapy I could to maximize the effects of my medication.

"I'm glad you're seeing good results," the new doctor told me.

"Yes, but I'm wondering what more I can do. I'm going to these therapy sessions. I exercise. I want to do everything I can to feel better."

"Well, a lot of people feel better on a low dose of thyroid medication."

"But—but my thyroid is normal, right? How would that make any difference?"

The doctor shrugged. "They don't know yet. But it helps a lot of my patients, even if their numbers are within the normal range."

The thyroid medication helped me, too. No one explained why. Life went on, and I felt almost normal for the first time since my teenage years.

When I got pregnant with my first child, my OB/GYN had a strict rule—no medications during my pregnancy. I did what she said and gave birth to a healthy baby girl. Allison. Postpartum, I couldn't get back on the right combination of meds. The doctor who prescribed the thyroid medication retired, and no one at his office would put me back on it. "Your numbers are normal," everyone said. Yet I could barely function. How normal is that?

Sixteen months after Allison was born, my dad got sicker. He'd had a chronic illness for as long as I could remember. We were close. So close. We fought our battles together, and now his was ending. That summer, Dad passed away. Time went on, and I tried to heal. My body refused. Even though I was grieving for my dad, I had a lot going for me. At every school where I applied for a teaching position, I received a job offer. My husband established his career, too. We had a beautiful, healthy family, a wonderful marriage, and financial security. Yet I still struggled.

Throughout the school year, I came down with chronic sinus infections. I missed a lot of work. It's hard to teach when you always need a sub. It's double the work to prepare lesson plans for a sub, then finish whatever the sub forgot. Sometimes I'd get lucky and get a good sub. A lot of times I didn't.

I felt hopeless. I didn't want to wake up in the morning. I didn't want to hurt myself, but I hated waking up and struggling through the day. So I took matters into my own hands. I read *everything* I could get my hands on. I tried every supplement that promised to give me some energy, if only for an hour or two. I talked with different doctors, I worked out harder, and I beat myself up when I couldn't. That didn't touch my pregnancy weight, which I still hadn't lost. So I restricted my calories. I tried to sleep "better" . . . yet I woke up every day feeling like I'd never been to bed at all.

When nothing else worked, I relied on caffeine. I've never been big on coffee, and energy drinks have too much sugar, so I developed a diet soda addiction. People warned me that I'd have trouble sleeping. I laughed. I could drink a twenty-ounce bottle of soda right before bed and fall asleep instantly. Every few months I'd get a wave of energy. I willed myself to work out more when this happened. Then the wave would crash, and my energy tanked again.

When I became pregnant with my second daughter, Olivia, my health got worse. Now that I was overweight, I'd developed high cholesterol. My thyroid numbers were still normal, yet I was told to take statins ("for life"). I slipped further into deep depression and debilitating fatigue. I felt like I had hit the lowest of the lows.

That's when I felt the lump. A literal lump in my throat. I could feel it when I swallowed. During my yearly checkup to get antianxiety meds, I asked my doctor to check it out.

"You feel that?" I asked as the doctor's cold fingers prodded my throat.

"Yes, right here. Hmm . . ." She felt around my neck. "And here."

I swallowed. Which was difficult.

"It's probably not a big deal," she said as she removed her gloves. "Ninety-eight percent of these lumps are benign. We'll do a routine test. I think it's caused by stress. Try not to worry about it."

But I knew it was cancer. I just knew.

The doctor scheduled an ultrasound, which didn't show anything. She referred me to a specialist with an eight-week-long waiting list. *No way. I want to see someone* now. Through a connection from my brother-in-law, I got an appointment that same week at the Mayo Clinic in Rochester. They did their own ultrasound and a biopsy.

Cancer.

This lump, of which 98 percent are benign, was thyroid cancer.

You get a diagnosis like that and you're in shock. Later that day, I heard that one of my classmates had just died of thyroid cancer. A girl I'd sat next to on the bus every day as a kid. A woman *my age.*

The cancer had taken over the right side of my neck and spread to several lymph nodes. What did that mean? I had a total thyroidectomy, lymphadenectomy, and radioiodine treatment to look forward to. Oh, and medication therapy. For the rest of my life. All the doctors and nurses told me this was the "best cancer to have," that treatment would be "easy," and that I was "lucky."

I scheduled the surgery and the radioiodine treatments. The radioactive iodine meant I had to separate myself from my kids. Radioactivity isn't good for little growing bodies. *Oh, yeah. This is the good kind. The easy cancer. I'm lucky to have this.*

The doctors told me that once I had the surgery and started my meds, I'd feel normal again. I hadn't felt "normal" in years. Would getting rid of this cancer be the secret to ditching my anxiety, depression, and fatigue?

Around the one-year anniversary of my diagnosis, I had a recurrence. More lymph nodes came back positive for cancer. Another surgery, more treatment. I watched tumor markers every four to six months. I had finally been prescribed thyroid medication again, and I had to take a higher dose to suppress my thyroid hormone—which also suppressed the cancer. The side effect of suppression was hyperthyroidism essentially (commonly known as an "overactive thyroid"), which brought even more symptoms. I was keeping cancer away at a high cost. Anyone who's ever tried to balance thyroid medications knows it's not easy. It's hard to feel normal. You don't look the same, you can't eat the same things, you don't have the energy to play with your kids, and you can't sleep. That's right—for the first time, I had trouble sleeping. There was nothing normal anymore. Not one thing.

I went back to the Mayo Clinic. I had to try something different.

"Is there anything I can do or take to help my symptoms?" I asked the doctor. "Because I'm not functioning here. I can barely make it to work. I can't sleep anymore. I can't take care of my kids. My husband travels a lot. I'm miserable."

"There's nothing else we can do. It takes time," he said. "Time is how we treat thyroid cancer." And then he added, "This is your new normal."

"I don't have more time to go on feeling like this. I have to be able to function. I've got these little people in my life. And I've got a career."

"I understand. What do you do?"

"I teach. High school."

"Ah."

I could tell he wasn't interested in helping me. I kept pushing anyway.

"It's not easy teaching high school kids. I need energy. I teach hard classes." I paused. My doctor said nothing. "If you won't help me, I'm going to find someone who will."

And I walked out.

That week in anatomy and physiology, I asked a student to read aloud a passage about the endocrine system. As she read, one sentence stood out.

"The thyroid gland affects every cell of the body."

I couldn't tell you how many times I'd taught that class, gone through that textbook, and read those same words. But I heard them now as if I was hearing them for the first time.

The thyroid gland affects every cell of the body.

And I no longer had one. Kind of a big deal, isn't it? I threw myself into more research, this time on the thyroid. I learned that it's not the thyroid itself but the thyroid hormone imbalance that causes depression, stress, anxiety, weight gain, muscle pain, blood sugar imbalances, everything. So how could I correct this imbalance? According to the doctors, my only hope was "time." My little spark of stubbornness or tenacity or whatever you want to call it made me search for something else, anything that could help me muddle through the day.

That thing was nutrition.

One Chance to Get Better

I've always been interested in the human body. My degree is in biology with a focus on human biology and microbiology. Even as a kid I was interested in nutrition and fitness. In college, I looked into the dietetics program, but it didn't feel right at the time.

One night after I put my girls to bed, I read an article that got me thinking about food. The author was a certified nutritionist. *Well, I eat pretty well, I think, but why not talk to an expert? I've got nothing to lose.* I don't know why that hadn't occurred to me before. The Mayo Clinic doctors focused on surgeries, medications, and treatment. They never mentioned nutrition beyond "just eat healthy" . . . whatever that means.

You see, I thought I knew what "healthy" food was. Turns out I didn't know anything. I was all about eating this many calories from these food groups. I thought if I drank a Diet Coke and ate fat-free SnackWell's it was a good day because I was keeping calories low.

I tracked down the author of that nutrition article. She was local, it turned out. I called her office and made an appointment.

This'll be different, I thought as I walked into her office. *She's not a doctor. She doesn't prescribe medications. Maybe this will be the answer.*

The room I was shown to looked more like a yoga studio than a doctor's office. I heard a light tap on the door. A tall, thin, smiling woman walked in to greet me.

"You must be Tiffany. What a pleasure to meet you!"

I felt intimidated. *What the hell could this happy, skinny, energetic woman know about fixing my problems?!*

"Yes, hello." I held out my hand.

"I see from your intake form that you're a cancer survivor. Congratulations."

If you can call this surviving. "Yes, thank you."

"And you're looking for ways to get your energy back?"

"Among other things. I've tried everything else," I said. Then I added, "You're my only hope!"

She chuckled. "Okay then! Why don't you tell me more about yourself. What are your goals?"

Just like that, the intimidation was gone. This lady had a super-sweet demeanor. I told her my story, and as we chatted, I found out she was also a farm girl from North Dakota. Like me. We went to the same university. She'd completed the same dietetics degree program that I had looked into.

"So what I'm saying is," I said, trying to wrap up my saga, "this is my one last chance to feel better."

"We'll get you feeling better." The nutritionist smiled at me. "I'm going to plug your symptoms and history into my program and tweak some things to fit your lifestyle. You'll leave today with a customized plan of what you should and shouldn't be eating every day."

"Custom? You mean, there's not just a standard, healthy diet I should follow? Eat fruits and vegetables every day and reduce my calories and all that?"

"Nothing about nutrition is standard. It's more about how the foods you eat nourish, heal, and support your body. And also identifying what you eat that detracts from your body. Your perfect foods are different than those of someone who doesn't have thyroid issues. This plan will be for your specific situation."

"Wow, that's more than I envisioned a dietitian doing. I've been doing fat-free and calorie counting. It's not working."

"Well, this isn't a 'diet.'" She tilted her head to the side. "This is functional nutrition. You're going to learn what nutrients do to support your body so you can feel better."

"Wow," I said again.

She opened her laptop. "Now, let's customize your plan."

I took that plan and her initial recommendations and put them into play. It wasn't too complicated. She basically had me do one thing—eat balanced meals. Proteins, fats, and carbs. Not fat-free. No calorie counting. Now, I didn't have diabetes, and I ate better than most of America, but I still had symptoms associated with imbalanced blood sugar. Needless to say I had a lot of room for improvement. Natural Lean Cuisines and fat-free potato chips aren't a balanced diet.

I cut out the worst culprits of my diet—the foods my nutritionist said were probably causing my brain fog, anxiety, depression, irritability, headaches, and swelling in my face, hands, and feet. I ate mostly whole foods instead. Within a few weeks, those balanced meals made a big difference. I started to feel level. Like myself. Balanced. Not hungry all the time. I had less brain fog. I had the energy to prepare healthy meals for me and my family. That was always sporadic before. I'd often relied on convenience over quality, taking the kids out for fast food. That was easier than planning, shopping, and standing in the kitchen chopping. But now I was actually *excited* to fix lunch for the kids. I couldn't remember the last time I'd been excited about anything.

I also got better socially. I didn't turn down party invitations anymore. I went to playgroups with my kids. I was more interested in the things I used to like. I worked out regularly like I used to, and it wasn't such a struggle.

I'd only changed one thing: I was eating balanced meals and snacks. From surviving to functioning to enjoying life again—all thanks to proper nutrition. When your goal is, "I just want to feel normal," and you don't even remember what normal is, there's nowhere to go but up. For me, each normal got better. I still had my ups and downs, but they weren't as bad as before. It felt like a miracle.

During my nutrition discovery, I struggled to do the job I had loved for so long—teaching anatomy and physiology. The classroom kept me stressed out.

"I'm still so exhausted," I told my husband one evening.

"You're doing so much better than you were," he said to me. "I see it in your face, your smile. And I hear it in reduced hits of the snooze button."

I laughed. "I know. I *do* feel better. I just . . . I think it's teaching. I must be burnt out or something."

"Time for a vacation? You could take a break from teaching."

"Maybe." I thought for a moment. "Maybe a permanent one."

I Want Her Job!

Visiting the nutritionist was the turning point in my well-being I needed. She'd handed me a map to better health, complete with clearly marked shortcuts. But something else happened, too. I didn't just learn about improving my diet. I also walked away thinking, *I want to be her. I want her job! I want to do what she does. I want to help other people find their own shortcuts to feeling better.*

If I had known three years earlier what I learned from her, I would've saved three years of my life. Three years of feeling better, functioning better, thriving, and enjoying life with my family. I knew I wasn't alone. There were other people in my situation. Maybe not the same diagnosis, but people who were fighting thyroid problems—maybe undiagnosed ones. And like me, they were struggling to find the energy to keep going. They didn't have to feel that way. I knew I could help them improve their health using what I'd learned about proper nutrition. I was sick and tired of teaching, so I used my newfound energy to go back to school.

In April 2014, I completed my master of science degree in human nutrition and performance (MSN). I also completed extra training and an internship to earn my nutritionist certification (CNS). So with my BS in biology, an MEd in education, an MS in nutrition, and a CNS, I started Rock Bottom Wellness, a nutrition consulting business where I teach proper nutrition to alleviate symptoms of thyroid issues. Why "rock bottom"? Because that's where I was when I found my nutritionist. That's where most of my patients are when they find me. In most cases, mainstream medicine drives us there.

Think about it. We go to the doctor and say, "I want to feel better." Then the doctor tells us how we're going to feel better—or *if* we're going to feel better. We let them dictate our outcome. We feel helpless. Maybe this medication or that treatment helps, but the side effects feel as bad as the underlying issue itself.

After years of being my own best advocate, I found my way up from rock bottom. Now I'm chasing my dream to help others find their way. At Rock Bottom Wellness, I help people improve their thyroid symptoms through proper nutrition education. My goal is to help people shortcut their path to living an amazing, healthy life and get to the root causes and underlying factors that affect people's day-to-day well-being.

I consider myself a thyroid expert in nutrition. When a client comes to me, we start with blood work. No, not the same blood work that your doctor orders. Instead of checking off boxes to see if you're "normal," I look for nutrient deficiencies. We fit nutrient-dense foods into your lifestyle to replenish those missing nutrients so you feel and function better. I *don't* tell you to eat 1,400 calories a day with three vegetables and two fruits. I look at the whole person, and together we come up with a practical plan specific to your needs. I also help you get your blood sugar in check while we manage your stress.

When I bring up thyroid hormone testing, my clients often say, "My doctor said I don't have symptoms, so he won't test it." Sound familiar? Even if you find someone willing to test your hormones, you end up having a version of this conversation:

You: Can I have my thyroid checked? I'm just so tired and down all the time. I thought you could look at it for me.

Doctor: Hmm . . . Have we had a sudden weight gain? Constipated? Puffy face?

You: No. I mean, I gained a little weight, but . . .

Doctor: That's to be expected at your age. Doesn't sound like a thyroid problem. Have you been under a lot of stress?

You: Maybe, but . . . could we just have it checked?

Doctor: That's really not necessary.

You: Please?

Doctor: (sighs) Okay, we can run your TSH.

Then at your next appointment . . .

You: So, what do my thyroid test results show?

Doctor: Let's see . . . here they are. Looks good . . . yes, all your numbers are in the normal range.

You: Oh. Well . . . good, I guess. If it's not my thyroid, is it something I'm eating? I try to eat healthy.

Doctor: You're fine; you're just getting older. Some fatigue is normal. Unless you have an allergy, the foods you eat don't have that much impact on how you feel. Try not to stress too much. I'll see you at your next physical.

What are your options at that point? Maybe you get a second opinion, but the new doctor tells you the same thing. Maybe you see a dietitian at the doctor's office. Doesn't help. You decrease calories and gain weight. You exercise more and feel worse. Then you look into alternative health care and buy some supplements that worked for your friend, your cousin, or your brother. You're ready to give up. But it's not over yet. Let me tell you about my client, Ray.

Ray has had type 1 diabetes since she was ten years old. When Ray came to me, she was tired. She had symptoms like aches and pains; headaches; red, blotchy skin; brain fog; and sudden weight gain. I noticed in her blood work there were indicators of another autoimmune condition. People with autoimmune diseases often have a gluten intolerance or gluten sensitivity. Rather than send her back to her doctor for expensive allergy testing, I told her to stop eating gluten for two months to see if she improved.

When you have diabetes, you have to take your insulin. That's all you can do, according to popular opinion. Everything else is out of your control. But Ray wanted her control back. I helped her take back that control through balanced eating and avoiding gluten. She lost forty pounds in eight weeks. Her skin cleared up. Her energy improved. She was able to start working out. We didn't drastically change her lifestyle, yet her health drastically improved anyway.

Another client, Darla, came to me with chronic, debilitating migraines. She'd seen a chiropractor and an acupuncturist for fourteen years. Their alternative therapies would help for a few days, but the migraines always returned.

"My chiropractor keeps saying I should come see you," Darla told me during our first appointment. "She thinks my migraines are systemic and can be fixed with nutrition. I keep telling her I already eat healthy." She sighed. "Well, I'll try anything. Maybe you can figure this out."

Darla followed my balanced eating recommendations. Within six weeks, her migraines were gone. She also lost ten pounds, even though weight loss wasn't her goal. Small changes, big difference. Oh, and Darla did all of this while traveling to Europe to visit family. She wasn't even at home in her own kitchen!

My client Judy was in her mid twenties when she found me. Judy had suffered from Crohn's disease–like symptoms since she was a teenager. She had severe gastrointestinal (GI) symptoms like cramping and blood in her stool. She was forty pounds overweight, and chronic fatigue kept her out of the gym.

At a recent appointment with her gastroenterologist, the doctor told Judy, "We need to put you on methotrexate."

I know methotrexate well. It's a chemotherapy drug with harsh side effects. For Judy, that was the last straw. She was going to grad school, she'd recently had a baby, and she knew she wanted to have more children.

"I'm too young to go on chemotherapy," Judy told me. "I want to lose weight, but I need to feel better first."

After our first appointment, Judy called her gastroenterologist.

"I'm going to give myself one year on this nutrition plan," Judy told her GI doc. "If it doesn't work, I'll go on your medication." Luckily, the doctor was on board. Judy followed my recommendations and lost thirty pounds in ten weeks. Her Crohn's symptoms disappeared—no more cramping or blood. No more fear of going out and not knowing where the bathroom is.

"I'm a new person," Judy told me.

I've worked with Judy for over a year now, and she's still not on methotrexate. And her gastroenterologist?

"Wow. Keep doing what you're doing."

So she does. Judy is thriving. So how did Judy (and Darla and Ray before her) lose weight? They didn't restrict their diet, obey "food rules," or complicate their family meals. They ate balanced meals, and weight loss just happened. That's what most of my clients experience. No one ever comes to me saying they need to lose X pounds. Symptoms first, weight loss second. With a classic dietitian, people go specifically to lose weight. But if you don't deal with the root cause, weight loss probably won't happen.

My client Steve could be described as tired and wired. He didn't sleep well. He had poor GI health. A lot of stuff in his life contributed to his symptoms—the loss of a parent, a divorce, and stress with his new stepfamily.

When Steve came to me, he told me, "I'm pretty calm. Things don't bother me."

I could see that. He had a passive demeanor with a calm presence. But when I looked at his nutritional testing, I saw nutrition deficiencies that correlated with stress. As I dug deeper, I saw that Steve *thought* he could handle anything. That wasn't true. He worked out too much for how he felt. Two hours a day, six days a week. We're talking intense activities like boxing and CrossFit. He never did calming exercises like yoga or meditation. In addition to a customized nutrition plan, Steve agreed to trade in a few of his boxing sessions for Pilates. When Steve went through my program, his anxiety and depression disappeared.

My client Jill came to me with chronic muscle pain, zero energy, and lots of frustration. She couldn't sit in one spot. She had to get up often to move around because of her pain. She couldn't sit at a restaurant and eat dinner with her husband after working all day.

Almost everyone who comes to me says they know how to eat well. But when we talk, they remind me of a young Tiffany—diet soda, fat-free chips, and maybe some carrots. Not Jill. Jill has what I call a high nutritional IQ. She was already adept at cooking healthy foods, but even so, she still struggled.

Jill completed my program in the midst of back-to-back travel for work and vacation. Her pain improved by 85 percent, and she lost ten pounds while working full-time at a desk job. As it turns out, even though she ate healthy foods, she was eating things that didn't agree with her. Her nutrient deficiency contributed to her symptoms, so that's what we focused on. As a result, she lost the inflammation that was causing her muscle pain. Now she can sit through a movie, she hikes, and she enjoys life.

When my client Harriet found me, she was depressed, overweight, and plagued with muscle and joint pain and insomnia. Her thyroid numbers were all over the place. Her husband had passed away suddenly, so she and her three kids were understandably a mess.

When Harriet went through my program, she started sleeping again. Rest gave her the energy she needed for her full-time job and her kids. She lost thirty pounds and went down a full shoe size thanks to decreased inflammation. Her depression lifted, and her muscle and joint pain subsided. By the end of the program, her thyroid numbers evened out.

I ran into Harriet at a live workshop recently.

"Tiffany, it's so good to see you," she said as she hugged me.

"You too, Harriet. You look amazing!" And she did. Her skin glowed, her hair shined, and her eyes brightened with joy.

"I feel amazing." She smiled. "Oh, hold on a minute, I want you to meet my friend." Her eyes scanned the crowd. Then she called out, "Jennifer! Come over here!"

A short, stout woman of about forty walked toward us.

"Tiffany, I want you to meet Jenn," Harriet said. "Jenn, this is the person who saved my life."

Another client, Lisa, was diagnosed with breast cancer ten years ago, and she beat it. This year, the cancer came back. It was in her lungs this time. Stage four.

"I know my chances aren't great, but I need to do a little more," Lisa told me. "I need to feel better. I need to not have pain. I need to support my treatment."

I wish everyone aspired to Lisa's positive outlook. Since completing my nutrition protocol, Lisa sleeps better. Her tumor markers have decreased. It's been a year since her regression, and she still has her energy. She's managing daily life well in spite of her diagnosis. Even if she's not cured, she's not going downhill anytime soon.

I'm always happy when my clients feel better. At the same time, I think, *What in the hell? This isn't rocket science. Why is this not a part of every person's health care process?*

Why isn't nutrition mainstream? Why do you have to work so hard to figure everything out through internet searches? Why is there a clash between mainstream medicine and nutrition? Why don't they go hand in hand?

My patients tell me they've tried to talk about nutrition with their doctors.

"Food doesn't affect how you feel," they say. "Food makes no difference. You're not taking supplements, are you? Those are dangerous!"

Maybe you're fortunate. Maybe you've found a doctor who's on board with certain vitamins. But when you ask questions, they may not know the difference between a professional-brand supplement and something off a drugstore shelf.

I don't expect doctors to know everything. Let's say you went to your family doctor with heart problems. They wouldn't make guesses about your treatment—they'd refer you to a cardiologist. They know you'd benefit from someone with special expertise. When it comes to nutrition, doctors receive little training in medical school or during residency. So why don't they refer patients to a nutritionist? Instead, many of them tell patients that nutrients don't matter and that people like me are selling snake oil.

If you or someone you love is struggling with a thyroid condition, the doctor probably said, "Here's your condition. Here's how you're going to go through this process. Here's how you're going to feel." When you asked when you could expect to feel normal again, they said, "You have a new normal now. Get used to it. Suck it up, Buttercup."

Frustrating, isn't it? I wasn't given any options either. I had to search for my own process. Now I want to share that process with you. If you're like many of my clients, you're undiagnosed, improperly diagnosed, or diagnosed and poorly treated. You feel sick. You're working, running your kids to their activities, and trying to hold your family together. You're guzzling coffee and faking it till you make it. Looking at you from the outside, no one would think anything was wrong with you. Inside, you're falling apart.

No more. In the chapters ahead, I'm going to help you:

- Stop just surviving and start thriving

- Balance your blood sugar

- Get off the mood roller coaster

- Diminish your cravings

- Sleep better

- Lose weight

- Lower your anxiety

- Give up food rules

- Navigate all the thyroid mumbo jumbo

- Advocate for yourself

- Feel better by using real nutrition

- Help your thyroid function optimally

- Believe there *is* something you can do to feel better

- Quit buying over-the-counter (OTC) supplements without knowing what you're buying or how they could affect your thyroid health

If you're struggling physically, mentally, or both, you have to be your own best advocate. I was stubborn enough to say, "I'm thirty years old. Don't tell me that this is my life. This sucks! I can't imagine this is why I was put on this earth."

I know it's hard. Especially when you're already feeling the lowest of lows in every way, shape, and form. I wrote this book to tell you that it *can* be better. It's not your fault you're struggling. The fact is you *can* feel better despite what you've been told. And you *will.*

R

CHAPTER 2

Eating to Feel Better Yesterday

"My personal nutrition and wellness had hit rock bottom, and I reached out to Tiffany with a plea for help. I had general knowledge about food, what is good for you, and what should be avoided, but my food habits did not demonstrate any understanding about the power of food. Tiffany has opened my mind and eyes. Our bodies are truly a machine, and what fuel is chosen is critical. I now have knowledge of what to look for. I have never felt so good physically and mentally."

— Keri L., Fargo, North Dakota

Whatever It Takes

When I was pregnant with my daughter Olivia, I was diagnosed with an eating disorder. It wasn't anorexia. Or bulimia. I've never starved myself or made myself throw up. My form of purging was a little different—I'm an exercise freak. Always have been. In college, I didn't walk on the treadmill after class. I *skipped* class for high-intensity interval training (HIIT). Some days I did two, three, even four HIIT workouts in a row. You're supposed to wait at least twenty-four hours between high-intensity sessions. I needed more energy to deal with my symptoms, and I hoped exercising would give it to me. It didn't. Yet I kept up my crazy exercise routine into adulthood—and motherhood. I exercised daily, most of the time, even though my body hurt all over. My depression made everything worse.

I finally healed my eating disorder through therapy during my second pregnancy. It felt good to clear my exercise obsession, but something else was wrong. Soon the lump would appear, and I'd be diagnosed with cancer.

When Olivia was a toddler, I scheduled an appointment with a functional medicine doctor to talk allergies. I don't mean hay fever. I went in to be tested for food allergies. Why not? I'd felt like crap for ten years. Maybe that gluten episode of *Oprah* was onto something. *If eating healthy isn't enough for me, maybe it's because I'm allergic to something!* The doctor tested me for dairy, gluten, egg, and soy antibodies. If my body didn't agree with any of these common food allergies, my immune system would show it on the test. I tested positive. For all four.

"This will be the key to improving your health," she told me. "But if you cheat, even occasionally, you won't see results."

I nodded solemnly. "Avoid the allergens. Got it."

"That's right. Dive into this one hundred percent. Don't eat anything with dairy, gluten, eggs, or soy. Make reading ingredient labels your new hobby."

I went a step further—it became my obsession. That restrictive diet triggered me. I went home and attacked the kitchen. Anything with dairy, gluten, egg, or soy, I threw into a box for the food bank or straight into the garbage.

"Help me get rid of all of them," I told my husband. "Read the ingredients labels. Closely. If I'm allergic to it, I want it out of here. I don't care how much it cost or how much we have left."

I probably sounded confident, but I felt afraid. Afraid to eat anything. I became hyperfocused and aware of food. I kept myself out of social situations like ladies' night out, playdates with other moms, and even dates with my husband. Or if I did go out, I just didn't eat. I was afraid to eat because I was afraid to feel like I had been feeling. My anxiety ramped up. It didn't matter. I needed to feel better yesterday.

I saw an internal medicine doctor for a second opinion, and he gave me horrible misinformation.

"You should just count calories. Eat one thousand calories per day."

"You mean . . . go back to eating dairy and everything? You don't think I'm allergic to them?"

"The science of allergy testing isn't settled. I see no reason why you shouldn't eat yogurt or bread. I'm confident your immune system is weak because you're overweight. Let's get that weight down first."

I may not have known what I know now, but I knew better than to starve myself. Undereating causes fatigue, hair loss, and skin disorders, all while wearing down your immune system so you get sick more often. Maybe this doc thought his "advice" would bring me back with symptoms he could write prescriptions for.

Another doc—my third opinion—was concerned about how much fluid I drank. She sent me to a specialist for diabetes insipidus treatment. *Crap, do I have this diabetes thing now, too?* I was scared, so I went. I'd always been thirsty my whole life. I was used to it, so it didn't seem like a huge concern. Even today I don't go anywhere without a reusable water bottle. But this third doctor expressed concern that my thirst meant something was deeply wrong. She couldn't tell me what. I found out later that there's a connection between thirst and thyroid function. Having thyroid cancer treatment fries your salivary glands so you feel thirsty all the time. You'd think one of these doctors would have made that connection.

I still followed every diet and exercise rule that the first doctor had given me. I also followed the USDA food pyramid (minus gluten and dairy). I wish I'd known how much lobbying went into the food pyramid so I wouldn't have fallen for it. I thought obeying the rules and avoiding the foods I was sensitive to would fix all my problems. For about two years, I kept every meal 100 percent free of gluten, dairy, eggs, and soy. This radical elimination diet was no fun—it started to help me feel better, and I was getting somewhere, but more had to be done because sustaining this extreme diet would be impossible to do forever.

So I stopped searching for new diets that did nothing. I had to try to forget everything mainstream medicine had taught me about nutrition. I had to get back to the basics. That's when I found the nutritionist who rocked my world. With her help, I started from scratch. I ditched all the rules about what I thought I should eat and when. You know the rest. It felt good to finally stop starting over.

Stop Starting Over

"I can't *not* have bread. There's just no way I can live without eating bread!" My new client grabbed her purse and stood up. "I have to have bread!"

"That's okay." I stood as well. "Many people are scared to death to remove a staple from their diet, whether that's bread, ice cream, or corn on the cob. Let's just deal with one thing at a time." I wondered if she was going to storm out of my office.

"Okay. Okay." She sighed and sat back down. "I'm sorry, I just—I just hear everyone saying I should give up gluten, and that's not gonna happen."

"Well, if you're diagnosed with celiac disease, of course you'll feel better when you stop eating gluten. But I don't think everyone needs to eat gluten-free. I *do* think that if you have a thyroid condition, you should be gluten-free."

My client nodded for the first time during our appointment. "Okay. So why is that, exactly?"

"Gluten is inflammatory, especially in large amounts. There's also a molecular mimicry with the protein molecule in gluten. Your immune system gets confused. It memorizes the structure of a foreign body and develops a defense to recognize it in the future. Being somewhat imperfect, your immune system attacks part of your own body along with the foreign invader. That basically means that your body thinks gluten is thyroid tissue, so it attacks your thyroid. No wonder gluten is one of the leading causes of autoimmune conditions."

"Oh, wow. I didn't know that."

"My point is, we're not short on reasons to cut back on gluten. I know it's hard. We think we need to have bread with our dinner. We're accustomed to our toast and pancakes. Whatever our ritual or tradition or culture, it's hard to imagine giving up something we've had our whole life."

"I've had bread with dinner for as long as I can remember. But if it's really making my body attack itself . . . I just . . ." She put her head in her hands. "I don't know what to do."

"I'll tell you one thing," I said. "I've seen people experience the most positive change when they understand where that change is coming from. If you're open to learning about what effect these foods have on you, you'll see a positive change, too."

"I am," my client said. "But what about when my husband and I go eat at his favorite Italian restaurant?"

"I'll help you learn to navigate situations like that," I said. "Sometimes, down the road, my clients are exposed to a situation where they don't have control over their food. They don't realize there's gluten hidden in their dessert. Or they're willing to risk a relapse for the warm, flaky biscuit everyone else at their table is having. They think, 'I'm going to eat this, and I know I'm going to feel horrible. I know it's going to happen, but I know how to get back to normal.' That's so much better than telling yourself, 'Oh my gosh, I feel terrible, I'm giving up.' That's the way life works. Take three steps forward, two steps back, then three steps forward, half a step back."

I'm telling you exactly what I told this woman—don't white knuckle it. Slowly transition. You need options and alternatives. "Don't eat anything with this, that, or those other things" is advice that doesn't work. You try it for a few weeks and feel miserable. Then you try something else you heard about from your best friend, mom, or social media. But that's not right for you either. Stop starting over. There *is* a way of eating that's realistic, practical, and right for you. We just don't know what we don't know.

Neither do a lot of health professionals. A lot of my clients have hired personal trainers before they came to me. When you want to lose weight and nothing else is working, why not pay someone to snap you into shape? Personal trainers often recommend high-intensity workouts because they supposedly give you faster results. That's not good for thyroid people. Then the trainer says, "Here's your nutrition plan. Go get all these supplements." Clients have brought me their list from their trainer. One *entire* piece of paper listing supplements to buy from GNC or Walmart. They have no idea what's in them or what they're for. The personal trainer probably doesn't either. They probably don't realize the negative impact they could have on someone with thyroid problems, someone on medication, or someone under adrenal stress. If you have thyroid issues, you go downhill quickly if you don't treat yourself carefully.

Instead of pursuing more knowledge and buying more stuff, what if you started getting only the *right* stuff? What if you learned what works for *you*? And what if you could reset your thyroid so you could feel better in a few short weeks?

The Rock Bottom Thyroid Reset: Feel Better in Eight Weeks

When I started my nutrition consulting business, I knew I couldn't put people through what I'd gone through. My clients were anxious enough already! Nowadays after a thyroid diagnosis, progressive doctors expect you to follow an extreme diet. I understand they're trying to help patients feel better. Better than hearing that what you eat doesn't matter! The problem is, it's expensive, it's hard, and it requires a lot of cooking. You have to inspect every ingredient like it's a crime scene. These diets are not sustainable, so they don't work. If life is nothing but crazy protocols for what you can and cannot eat, it's hardly worth living. There *is* a different way. One that works. A plan that's all about starting simple, collecting some easy wins, and building up from there.

The Rock Bottom Thyroid Reset teaches you the basics of eating to feel better—and lets you forget about everything else. Why name this reset (and my business) Rock Bottom? Because that was me. *I* hit rock bottom. Nowhere to go but up. The people I met down there are the people I want to help. If you've hit your rock bottom or if your thyroid is taking you there, the Rock Bottom Thyroid Reset is for you.

But is my protocol the *best* plan for you? You have your choice of over three thousand books on thyroid health alone. Not to mention the forty thousand books on healthy, balanced eating. Why is the Rock Bottom Thyroid Reset any different? Because more information and more knowledge isn't going to help get you results. If all it took to ditch depression, feel energized, and drop the pounds was learning more about gluten, you wouldn't need this program. You would google "gluten-free bread near me," and your whole life would magically change.

I had that information. I had the education about biology, biochemistry, and nutrition. Then there were all the thyroid facts I looked up online. I read the bestselling diet books. Everything felt daunting. The more I learned, the less I wanted to do. So many rules to follow. So much anxiety. *Screw that . . . I can't do this!*

When I hit rock bottom and didn't know what else to do, I had to figure it out. You know what I discovered? People like us need a shortcut. Not more information. Not an endless supplement list. Not recipes that take four hours to make. We need a practical plan designed for our hectic life. We need simple tips and quick wins. And we need to understand the root causes of our thyroid symptoms so we can stop comparing ourselves to others.

I hear all the time, "Well, my sister did this," and, "My mom followed this diet." Maybe that worked for them, but you're in a different situation. Your biochemistry is different than theirs. With my program, you get to skip boring nutrition class and the internet search rabbit hole of bad advice. Go straight to feeling better!

So how does the Rock Bottom Thyroid Reset work? It's simple and short—two weeks for preparation, two weeks for repair, and then it's time to rebuild.

In the first phase—the prep phase—our objective is to decrease your inflammation. We'll prepare tasty whole-food snacks and meals, improve your gut health, balance your blood sugar, and manage your stress. Clients tell me they feel like a new person two weeks later.

Then during the two-week repair phase, we're going to balance your hormones to repair your thyroid. How? You'll do some detoxing so your liver can help convert your thyroid hormones better. Nothing crazy that will keep you chained to the bathroom for three days. Think of it like cleaning house. We'll get rid of extra junk holding you back—hormones, toxins, chemicals. That's the core of the reset. Then we start back at zero.

In Week Five and beyond, you'll rebuild your energy and your mood for lasting health. We'll add foods back in, testing to see how they make you feel. You'll be able to self-guide your food choices long-term based on how your body responds.

The reset is flexible. If you need two weeks or even a month to complete "Week One," that's how long you take. You should be able to follow the program and go along with your life rather than forcing yourself to stick to it. If you cram in too much too fast, it's not going to last.

Some new clients tell me, "I can't start your program until my vacation is over," or, "I need to wait until after Christmas before doing the reset thing." It's true—you shouldn't detox on a fourteen-day cruise. That doesn't mean you can't begin working through your issues. When people start the Rock Bottom Thyroid Reset and see how certain foods make them feel, they can enjoy the vacation, the holidays, and everything else. They better navigate tough situations like parties and vacations because they've paid attention and understand their body.

That said, you're probably eager to put the reset into play. Before we prep your body so you can feel better in every possible way, we have to prep your mind. Why get your head in the right place first? Because I don't want to set you up for failure. If you're jumping into a program out of desperation but aren't open to making changes, you're not going to do well. Some people think these changes are drastic. Honestly, if you're ready to climb out of your rock bottom, the changes won't be an issue.

At a business networking event the other day, a man asked me, "Tiffany, what do you do if someone wants to lose weight and have more energy, but they don't want to change what they're eating?"

I was pretty blunt. "Well, I'd tell the person I can't work with that. You can't have it both ways. Either you want to improve your life or you don't."

"Yikes." The guy shuffled his feet. "That takes a lot of nerve. Plus you'd lose the person as a client."

"Actually, people *have* said that to me. I simply let them know they're not my people. As far as losing their business, you can't lose what you don't have. There's no point in deceiving people, letting them think they can pull off a magic trick with their health. Wouldn't you agree that honesty is the best policy?"

He mumbled something affirmative and excused himself to the donut table.

I'm not going to deceive you either. If you want to reset your thyroid so you can do things that make you feel like you again, you have to embrace change. I'm not talking about change for the sake of change. "Eat this, not that, because the nutrition lady said so." No, I'm going to be right here with you, showing you why we're doing what we're doing and making lasting change as easy as possible. The Rock Bottom Thyroid Reset is the shortcut you've been looking for.

Our first stop is the space between your ears.

R

CHAPTER 3

Think Right, Feel Better

"My A1C went down to 5.6 percent! This means I am no longer pre-diabetic! The doctor said whatever we are doing is working, so keep it up. Thank you, Tiffany!"

— Brandy R., Youngstown, Ohio

"I saw a naturopath a few months ago, and I already have a meal plan to get my thyroid and everything back on track. I can follow it myself," someone at a business networking event told me after I introduced myself. She said nothing about herself or her business. Just a clear "I don't need what you do." People can be so friendly, can't they?

If you could do this all by yourself, you would've done it by now. There's no reason not to get your body working right, and you still haven't done it.

At Rock Bottom Wellness, I see a lot of people put off their health. A new client learns about the Rock Bottom Thyroid Reset. Then she says, "Great, I'll get back to you about starting after the holidays . . . after my birthday . . . after vacation."

Why the resistance to eating and feeling better today? Now? Why wait? I blame the hard and restrictive diets we're used to following.

Remember the "whole thirty" plan? It has you avoid all soy, dairy, grains, alcohol, legumes, and added sugars for thirty days. I can't tell you how many times people tell me something like, "I already know about eating well. I've done that whole-foods thirty-day thing. But I can't do that forever. It was so overwhelming!"

The Rock Bottom Thyroid Reset is the opposite. You don't need the courage to cut your daily calorie intake in half. And you don't need to pump yourself up with daily affirmations to feel motivated to stick with it. If you want to feel better, you need fast results. I get it. That's what I designed my program to do. Get quick wins, and you meet your need for motivation. I've built motivation into the program! For example, you change a couple of things in the first week. You start feeling better, so you *want* to keep doing them. You're not starting a radical diet where you feel worse the whole first week. With my program, you start getting little wins right away—then you have a reason to keep the ball rolling. All those little wins snowball into bigger wins.

Sounds too simple, doesn't it? The secret to earning small victories that change your life is your mindset. Shift your expectations about everything a diet should be and you set yourself up to feel better sooner than you thought possible.

Six Mindset Shifts to Get Fast Results

Here are six simple ways to shift your mindset so you make the most of your thyroid reset efforts.

Think Outside the Pyramid

Remember learning about the food pyramid in elementary school? You probably had to memorize the six food groups—grains, veggies, fruit, dairy, meat and legumes, and sugary, fatty junk food. Remember the quizzes on putting different foods into the right category? Maybe you even had to hand-make your own pyramid for the science fair.

Since then you've heard more variations on that pyramid than you can remember. Atkins, paleo, keto, vegan, gluten-free, low-carb, slow-carb, low-fat, high-fat. Every article promises perfect health from the hot new diet. How can you even tell what's healthy anymore? Or maybe you've never taken fad diets seriously. I come from a town where everybody eats meat and potatoes (or hotdish or casserole). The menu never changes. Either way, I'm not going to suggest you cut out carbs or fats. Nothing drastic. Instead, we're going to talk about balanced eating and whole foods.

It can be hard to wrap your head around switching from the standard Western diet to whole foods, even if you know McDonald's cheeseburgers and Hungry-Man frozen dinners are far from healthy. The first step toward improving your health is to be open to different foods you may never have tried before.

"I'm already eating healthier," a new client told me. "And I know how to do low-carb for weight loss."

She threw out more bits of knowledge, as if to prove she didn't need my advice.

"I can tell you've read a lot about food and health," I finally said. "But not every diet is right for every person, no matter how popular it is. Even if you know all the right foods you should be eating, knowing what we *should* do isn't always enough. When it comes down to it, what we *actually* do doesn't always live up to our own expectations. That's why I want us to create a personalized plan that you can easily stick to."

"But I'm already doing all the right things. I just don't understand why I feel like crap!"

I stopped sugarcoating it. "Honestly, I don't think you *could* feel good eating what you've been eating. And you won't feel better doing what you're doing. If you always do what you've always done, you're going to get what you've always gotten. You have to be open to changing what you put in your body."

She was silent for a minute. "Fine. What's my personalized plan?"

Everyone's plan looks different because everyone's body is different. But the basis for everyone's diet should be whole foods.

But I'm a picky eater. How is this food going to taste?!

First of all, I'm not asking you to eat plain, boiled brussels sprouts or to put kale in everything. Prepared right, whole foods are delicious. When you start cooking real food and reducing processed foods, something else happens. Your taste buds *change*. You start to have more of an affinity for healthier foods. The donut doesn't sound as appealing as it once did. When you give your body what it needs, it starts to ask for more. Before you know it, you'll be thinking, *Gosh, broccoli sounds good right now.*

"I like mac and cheese, I like cold cut sandwiches, and I eat at the diner a lot," another client once told me. "I want to change . . . but I'm not looking forward to it. I just don't know where to start."

"Okay, what meal is the hardest for you?" I asked. "Out of breakfast, lunch, or dinner, where are you most dreading change?"

"Probably breakfast. I don't know what I'd do without my sausage biscuit."

"Great," I said. "Let's focus on breakfast first. We'll establish some good, nutritious, doable meals for breakfast. Forget about the rest for a little while. Taking one step at a time helps you set yourself up for success. Once you get those down and you feel comfortable, we'll move on to lunch."

"I'm pretty rushed in the morning. How long are these meals gonna take? And what if I don't like them?"

"I'll make sure they're practical *and* tasty. And you can call me and let me know what you think."

My client called me the next day.

"So I gave that first recipe a try."

"Yeah? What did you think?"

"Well, I'll tell you, I wasn't looking forward to it . . . but . . . I guess it doesn't taste bad after all. It wasn't hard to make either. Didn't take much longer than waiting in line at the drive-through for my biscuit."

"I'm glad to hear that."

"But the real reason I'm calling you," he said with a sigh, "is because this is the first morning in a while I'm not falling asleep at my desk."

"That's because you've eaten something that doesn't make you crash and burn."

"Yeah, no crash today. So when do I start working on lunch?"

When you give people permission to start small, they set their own tone for more progress. Breakfast is the first place I started, too. The biggest breakthrough for me was learning that I didn't have to have "breakfast food" for breakfast. You can eat anything for breakfast. You can eat dinner for breakfast! Back in the day, there were no Froot Loops. There were no donuts. Just because these foods are being marketed as breakfast foods doesn't mean you have to eat them. You can have leftover vegetables from the night before and throw in an egg. You don't need pancakes or cereal. When you don't eat sugary or high-fat foods in the morning, you feel better the rest of the day. You set yourself up for success rather than crashing and cravings.

A family friend told me that her seven-year-old once asked for leftover turkey and sweet potatoes.

For breakfast.

"Oh my gosh, that's crazy! You can't have that for breakfast," her mother told her.

"Why not?" she asked.

"You should have toast or cereal," her father said. "Or we can make pancakes."

"Yes," her mother said. "But you can't have turkey and potatoes for breakfast."

But turkey and potatoes was what she wanted. Her body needed protein and complex carbs. At seven years old, she already knew how to listen to her body instead of TV commercials. The rest of us have forgotten how.

Be Open to Learning

I recently attended a women's business conference. In one session, the presenter taught how to increase your conversion rate on consult calls. *Sell my services over the phone? I'm already great at that!* I thought. When I offer people a free consultation call, 85 percent end the call as a client. That's because most prospects either follow me online or hear about me from a mental health therapist or chiropractor. By the time I talk to future clients, they've already been warmed up to me.

A free consult call usually goes something like this:

"So, what's bothering you?" I ask. "What are your main health concerns right now?"

"I'm always tired and in pain. When I wake up in the morning, my joints ache. When I get home, my back hurts. I never have the energy to do the things I know I should be doing, and I feel stuck."

"What do you want to change, and how do you want to change it?"

"I want to feel good again! I want to stop hurting all the time. I've already tried physical therapy, and I go to a chiropractor. I want to try eating differently."

"What's stopped you in the past from changing your diet?" I ask.

"I guess I was just too overwhelmed . . . I don't know where to start."

I identify their pain points; then I offer them a mini plan. I give my impressions plus some things they can do short-term.

"After hearing about your pain, I think you might have some form of an autoimmune disorder," I say. "My gut feeling is that you should cut back on sugar to decrease your inflammation. And because you're so tired, your thyroid might not be functioning properly. So I'd also try avoiding gluten to see if that gives you more energy."

Then I suggest the plan I feel is right for them. I see how they respond, and we go from there. Not much to improve on, right?

Anyway, back to the business conference. I took a seat in the back row for the session. I wasn't expecting to learn anything. *Please, I could* teach *this.* I got out my laptop to work on my email newsletter and caught this Claude Bernard quote in my notes:

> *It's what you think you already know that*
> *prevents you from learning.*

Well . . . okay . . . maybe there's something I could improve on.

You don't know everything, no matter how familiar you are with something. I hear all the time, "I already know how to do that."

That's why I'm asking you to be open to learning. Even if you think you already know everything there is to know about nutrition. Ever heard of the marketing rule of seven? It's shorthand for the idea that your customers need to see your advertisement at least seven times before they buy. The same applies to nutrition. If you see a message like "avocados are healthy" seven times, you remember to add them to your shopping list. Introduced a new food to your kids lately? They hate that bite of broccoli the first six times. Then the seventh time, they say, "Oh, I guess I like that." When you're open to new foods, your body receives them with open, well, open taste buds!

Keep It Family-Friendly

People call me because they need help. Most have families. That's why I help my clients make their food a part of family life. This isn't "your food" where you get takeout for everyone else. I don't recommend that anyway. Sustainable, healthy eating benefits spouses and kids, too.

What if your partner raises his eyebrows? What if your teenager turns up her nose? Be strong. Tell your family, "This is how we're eating now. It's going to make us healthier and stronger, and it's going to taste good, too!" You can adjust most recipes so everyone enjoys them. Pass your partner some hot sauce, get out the gluten-free crackers for yourself, and add a banana on the side for your toddler. You don't have to make a separate meal to satisfy everyone. Variations of the same meal don't have to be time-consuming or difficult.

Not everyone is going to like every food. And not every new food is going to come out perfect. I remember when I first tried to make banana bread with different types of flour. More than one loaf ended up squirrel food in the backyard. But foods like vegetables and other staples weren't an issue at all. Add seasoning and spices, get used to cooking with fresh food, and everything you prepare is full of flavor. Your family might not even realize you're not serving them junk anymore.

Teach Your Body What You Don't Need

The Rock Bottom Thyroid Reset is a progression. It's a process, not an extremist diet. But there may come a time when you need to be firm. You may need to stay away from a certain food—at least for a month - maybe longer. Even if you have to white knuckle it. Why a month? That's how long it can take to get certain foods out of your system. Then you can see how you feel when you add it back into your diet. Think of it as a tool to learn how foods do or don't affect you. Sometimes you have to go cold turkey on certain things for a short period of time to retrain your body.

When I say "certain things," most people think gluten. Often, dairy is the problem. Dairy is addictive. I've had clients who eat ice cream every night. Their nose runs constantly. What happens when they switch to almond ice cream? Sinuses clear up. The downside? It only works if you eliminate *all* dairy. Sometimes you can't do moderation. I hate that word anyway. It's not realistic. Addicted people can't moderate an addiction.

How do you know if *you* have a food addiction? Ever find yourself saying, "I need this food"? That's probably a food addiction. Typical food addicts feel like they need a food until they stop eating that food and start feeling better. That's when they don't want the food anymore. Addiction, broken. That's the breakthrough, not only for people who feel like they need a certain food but also those of us with pesky cravings. This thyroid reset plan ties what you're eating to how you feel. Then if a situation arises where that food is in front of you, and you eat it because you freaking want it, you know what results to expect. You also know how to move past it. (Need one-on-one help breaking a food addiction? My six-month hold-your-hand version of the Rock Bottom Thyroid Reset incorporates emotional-eating supportive education.)

"You mean if I tell you I know I'm going to feel like crap if I eat this, but I'm going to eat it anyway, you're not going to yell at me?!" One client looked at me with disbelief. We discussed her and her partner's anniversary cheesecake tradition. "I'm going to eat it *even though* I know what the consequences will be, because it's worth it to me at that time. If I do that, you're not going to lecture me?"

"No, I won't yell at you. I won't quietly judge you. Because you can fix it starting right after your meal."

I know a couple of people who've gone through some life events and fallen off the wagon, so to speak. But they know what they can do to get back on. When they do, they say, "Wow! *That* was what was making me feel so bad." It's never too late—or too early—to show your body what it doesn't need.

Remember That Some Days Are Better Than Others

Once you figure out what's causing your symptoms, the healing process can start. As you move into Week One of the Rock Bottom Thyroid Reset, you might think, *I can't keep doing this through Christmas!* Or, *What about my birthday?* Or, *We're going to have to cancel our vacation.* Some people quit. They give themselves an excuse. They go back to what they know, what they're comfortable with, what they want. And they undo what they've done because they think it's all or nothing.

I'm telling you it's not. It's not always easy to ride the craving waves, but stick with the plan and you'll feel your best the longest. If you look at your calendar for the year, you'll find at least twelve excuses to say, "Screw it." So could I. But if I'd said "screw it" every time a special occasion came up, I never would've progressed. You have to power through. If you have a crappy day of eating crappy food, oh freaking well! Start over the next day or the next hour or the next minute.

It's like hiking up a winding mountain trail. You feel like you're going backward sometimes, but you're still moving uphill. Sometimes it will seem high. If you stumble back, you can keep going forward. You don't have to *stop* feeling better.

My husband does this thing every January. We always laugh about it. Everybody makes fun of him for it. Sometimes that includes me. Every January, he doesn't drink any beer.

"I can't *not* drink beer," his friends say. "The Super Bowl is coming up. And then it's my birthday, and then it's my wife's birthday, and then . . . there's just no way I could give up beer. No way."

"Okay, then pick a different month," my husband says. His buddies go through their whole year but can't pick one month to give up alcohol. If that's your mindset, you're never going to change—or feel better. There will *always* be a reason not to.

But what if you remembered the reasons why you should? What if instead you asked, "How do I make my life fit into this program?" Healthy eating shouldn't be a special thing that you're either on or off. It's just part of your life. As the years have moved on through his yearly tradition, those who have thought it would be impossible for them have not done their own versions of clean eating/less beer drinking in January.

See Beyond Good and Bad

I hear people in day-to-day conversations say, "Oh, I'm going to be bad today. I'm going to have french fries." Why is that bad? Because french fries are unhealthy? Who cares? If you want some freaking fries, have some fries! When you start making changes, you'll find the fries (or other deletable food) not that great or appealing anyway.

I've never claimed to be a perfect eater—whatever that is. I don't give food power over me. I give the power to what my body needs. Don't label a food good or bad so you can use it as an excuse. *Well, I ate something bad, so screw it. I'll eat bad the rest of the day. What's the difference now?*

On the flip side, some people think unhealthy foods are "good."

How do you get your calcium if you don't drink milk? There's no other way! You don't need to drink dairy to get calcium. Dairy can cause all kinds of health problems. Instead, try leafy greens, sesame seeds, legumes, or tofu. We'll talk more about those foods soon.

Now you're beginning to see what sustainable, healthy eating looks like. You know the hardest part is adjusting your mindset and committing to the right path. Even if you stumble. You also know it doesn't have to be the end of ice cream or cheesecake (even though I'm going to ask you to avoid both for at least thirty days).

You're excited. You're nervous. You're committed to feeling better, and you're ready to learn how.

Let me show you where to start.

R

CHAPTER 4

Rock Bottom Thyroid Reset: Phase One

"I was starting to feel my age. I no longer feel that. Overall, I am so excited for how much better I can feel! This is amazing. No dairy, no gluten, no grains, no sugar. I have followed this for about a week. I can feel the inflammation leave, and my blood pressure has been level."

— Ken F., Minneapolis, Minnesota

The Preparation Phase: Two Weeks to Feeling Good

The Rock Bottom Thyroid Reset will help you eliminate problem foods, get back to the nutrition basics, and make you feel like yourself again. During the Preparation Phase—your first two weeks on the protocol—we'll get rid of the junk in your diet. Now, before you panic, remember that a lot of these changes are temporary. We need to drop certain foods, then gradually add them back in to see if they're a problem for you. Even if some foods are an issue long-term, you're still not saying goodbye forever to anything that's not a vegetable. If something you eat makes you feel terrible, we can find substitutes you enjoy instead (more on alternatives to your favorites later). For now, we're going to keep things basic.

During Week One, I'm going to help you remove gluten from your diet. During the second week, we'll remove dairy. During both weeks you'll replace fried, fatty, sugary foods with whole, nutritious, tasty foods that make you feel good—and good about yourself.

But I Thought "Gluten-Free" Was a Fad Diet?

If you struggle with a thyroid condition, you want to stay away from gluten. Gluten causes inflammation, which is associated with autoimmune disease. And as you know, your thyroid functions as part of your immune system. It's so easy to let that cycle send your health in a downward spiral, which is why it's best to avoid gluten altogether.

If you have a thyroid issue, you're also more likely to have what's called "leaky gut." This is when your small intestine (which absorbs nutrients from your food) becomes too permeable, or "leaky." Instead of moving through your digestive tract, small particles of food flow into your bloodstream. Pretty scary, isn't it? Eating gluten contributes to leaky gut, causing the cells in your intestinal wall to open up. When this happens over and over (think bagels for breakfast, pasta for lunch, pizza for dinner), you're set up for poor gut health. You can't absorb nutrients, you get constipated, and you may even develop acid reflux/GERD (gastroesophageal reflux disease). In short—eat gluten, get sick.

Okay . . . So What Can I Eat?

Real food. As much as you can, you want to eat organic, unprocessed whole food. For meat, eat grass-fed whenever possible. This way your liver can get a break from processing so many chemicals and hormones. If money or accessibility make this difficult, do the best you can. Frozen chicken breast beats frozen TV dinners. Make *better* choices, not *perfect* choices. You'll still feel the benefits, even if you're 75 percent of the way there. Two weeks from now, you'll be eating both gluten-free and dairy-free, and your diet will consist of whole, balanced foods. Two weeks from today, you can expect:

● Increased energy and vitality

● Weight loss and reduction in body fat

● Healthier skin and softer hair

● More restful sleep

● Clearer thinking and a happier mood

● Healthy habits established for improving your health long-term

● Emotional stability

● Fewer cravings

● No blood sugar plunges

● Reduced sleepiness during the day

● No more headaches

Maybe you're trying to lose weight. If so, excess body fat might not be your problem. The heaviness you're feeling is probably due to excess fluid and inflammation. After Week One, you're going to feel lighter. Your feet won't hurt every morning when you put them on the floor. Your wedding ring will fit better. Your eyes will stop watering. You won't annoy people with sniffles and throat clearing.

I hear stories like these all the time. My client Jane hated grocery shopping. She hated doing the laundry. She dreaded every mundane task because she was so tired. After the first week of the Prep Phase, her life started to normalize. The tasks and chores she'd hated for so long weren't a big deal anymore.

Jane had never been into working out, but now she had more energy and more stamina—both mental and physical. She felt herself getting stronger. For the first time in her adult life, she could get the benefits of regular exercise—all because she changed her diet. Now, Jane wasn't doing HIIT workouts or living in the gym all day. She enjoyed afternoon walks, evening yoga classes, and weekend bike rides with the kids. She didn't overdo it by trying to burn a ton of calories. Her consistent exercise became more effective as she continued to balance her blood sugar with simple meals. She was fueling her body with things that contributed to her health versus things that took away from it.

Before my client Brad found me, he was so tired he needed a cup of coffee before he could even get ready for work in the morning. Then he'd have another cup on the way. He was still tired once he got to work, so he'd often grab a third. Of course he never had time to pack a decent lunch, and he didn't take time for breakfast. Every single day, Brad started behind the eight ball.

In the first two weeks of following the Rock Bottom Thyroid Reset, Brad balanced his blood sugar by eating simple whole-food meals. Now, instead of three cups of coffee, one was plenty. Some days he forgot to drink it at all! He stopped falling asleep on the way to work. He felt more focused, and he could stay on task longer.

Maybe you can relate to Jane and Brad. Or maybe your mornings are decent but your energy and focus take a huge dip in the afternoon. That was my client Sarah. Every day right around two or three in the afternoon, the only thing she wanted was a nap. She felt hopeless. Like she'd never be able to get through the day. There are some natural rhythms in your body that dip toward the end of the workday. That doesn't mean you should need to set up a bed underneath your desk! When you balance your meals, you balance your blood sugar and manage stress better. Then you don't crash in the afternoon. You don't need to take a nap or look for cake, cookies, and coffee in the break room to get you through the rest of the day.

Like many of my clients, Sarah was skeptical that cutting out gluten and dairy would help her. Since her best friend had lost fifteen pounds, Sarah had been following a cottage cheese diet with her. Sarah was also worried that she wouldn't have the willpower to follow my program. But she was at her rock bottom and willing to try anything. Within the first two weeks, Sarah went from cloudy, moody, and depressed to hopeful, positive, and energetic.

"You know, I can do this," Sarah told me on the phone. "I don't know what I was so scared of. This isn't so bad. I'm starting to feel better. I have more energy. I can focus. I can play with my kids. My body doesn't feel so puffy. And not only that, I have a better outlook now. I can do it! I can live and thrive instead of being a putz."

Once Sarah started earning these little wins, she felt empowered.

"I learned something about my body this week, and I'm in control of it," Sarah told me once dairy was out of her diet. "I'm feeling better because of what I'm doing for myself, not because I'm copying what worked for someone else."

You may think the only purpose of this Prep Phase is to take stuff out of your diet. It's also a time to become aware of your body, to listen to what it's saying, and to make a conscious choice to give it what it desires. You don't have to let someone else predict the outcome of your health and well-being. That's why I hate it when doctors recommend calorie counting. You'll see calories listed in the Prep Phase meal ideas sections because I don't want you to go too *low* on calories. But there's no need to calorie count—you have an innate ability to listen to your body. You just have to remember how.

Will I Go Broke Changing My Diet?

Some people have sticker shock when they see the price of gluten-free bread. *Oh my gosh, it's eight dollars a loaf! And it's half the size of a regular loaf!* Gluten-free bread isn't a necessity. Nor is most of it even that healthy. Yet it does help a lot of people transition their eating habits. When you've had bread with dinner for the last twenty years, it's much easier to have a substitute than to give bread up entirely.

People always think eating healthy is expensive. Gluten-free bread aside, that's often not the case. It all depends on what you're buying. When you buy eggs and baby spinach to make one of my breakfast meal ideas, you realize that eating well doesn't have to eat a hole in your wallet. There are more expensive healthy foods just like there are more expensive junk foods. When you're buying crackers, cookies, and other processed boxed foods, the grocery bill adds up. It's expensive in two ways—for your body and your bank account. The next time you meet a friend for coffee, skip the macchiato and opt for an Americano. You'll avoid a blood sugar spike, *and* it's half the price of a fluffy sugary drink!

While some healthy foods are a little pricier than their junk food counterparts, the majority of what you'll buy during the next two weeks is affordable. You're not eating exotic gourmet foods. We're all about balanced eating.

I've been trying to convince a friend of mine to start eating simple meals. Every hour she says something like, "Oh my gosh, my blood sugar dropped. I need to eat something. Oh my gosh, I need some protein." All day long.

"Eat an actual whole meal, not just chips and soda!" I tell her. I bet you she eats ten times a day because her blood sugar drops nonstop. After this many years, she's probably headed for a diabetes diagnosis. But it's never too late to start eating balanced meals. One day I'll convince her.

So What Exactly Is Balanced Eating?

When I say balanced eating, I'm referring to balancing the macronutrients like proteins, fats, and carbohydrates. When first starting my program, people often need to eat balanced meals several times a day to get back on track. After a few weeks, their mood swings and plummeting blood sugar even out, and eating two or three meals a day becomes comfortable.

This is why the Rock Bottom Thyroid Reset meal plans include a full serving of proteins, carbohydrates, and fats at each meal (and half that at snacks). You can modify each meal idea to fit your needs and maintain satiety (i.e., feeling full instead of hungry). I don't want you to starve yourself! Let's keep cravings at bay. Most people who have symptoms of imbalanced blood sugar do best with three meals and two snacks a day for a couple of weeks. As your hunger decreases, you can eliminate snacks if you like. I have this laid out for you over the next six weeks, but you can extend the plan as long as you need. Remember, the goal is to balance your blood sugar and manage your stress while supporting your thyroid.

Are Carbs Good or Bad?

Both, depending on the type! When we choose whole-grain, veggie, or fruit carb sources, we don't develop the health problems associated with processed carbs. That said, we need to watch what carbohydrates we're putting into our bodies. It doesn't matter if the food is sweet or not—if it's a carb, your body will convert it to sugar. Some carbohydrates turn into more sugar faster than others. Whether you eat a glazed donut, a bowl of Cheerios, or a cup of broccoli, it turns into sugar. But look at the difference:

3/4 cup Cheerios – 6 teaspoons of sugar

1 cup broccoli (raw) – 0.92 teaspoons of sugar

If you transition to getting your carbohydrates from whole foods, you'll feel so much better in so many ways. Rock Bottom Thyroid Reset meals are designed with balance in mind. When you balance your macronutrients, you have better blood sugar stability. That means you'll feel less irritable and less anxious. If you're mindful of that as you go through your day, you'll make better carbohydrate choices. What does it mean to be mindful? Well, I'm going to show you how to pay attention to the types of foods you're eating. As you make food choices throughout your day, keep this simple formula in mind:

Total grams of carbohydrates divided by 4 = number of teaspoons of sugar your body converts those carbs into

For example: 28 grams carbohydrates $\div$ 4 = 7 teaspoons of sugar

You don't have to obsess over this formula. It's just another way to be mindful about the amount of sugar you're taking in on your whole-food eating journey. We're often led to think that because we're eating a bunch of whole grains, we're not eating too much sugar. People think "sugar" means something sweet like candies, cookies, and doughnuts. Of course, avoiding sweets will reduce your sugar intake. But we also need to think of the other carbohydrates that turn into sugar in our body. Most of us don't connect the dots between a potato and the sugar it turns into. To give you the gist of it, here's a brief lesson on how food turns to sugar.

When you eat food, whether it's sweet or not, your body converts it into glucose (sugar) and uses it for energy. Let's look at three common foods. First, skim milk. One cup of skim milk has twelve carbohydrates, which converts to three teaspoons of sugar. Second, let's look at corn chips. A serving size of twenty-one chips converts into four and a half teaspoons of sugar. And let's be realistic—most people don't eat just twenty-one chips when they're at a party or making nachos. Third, let's look at Cheerios. Plain Cheerios, not honey nut or sweetened varieties. Three quarters of a cup of Cheerios equals six teaspoons of sugar. Often cereal is marketed as wholesome and good for you. Like other common breakfast foods, most cereals are highly processed. Combine these with skim milk and orange juice—a "complete breakfast"—and you're getting a lot of sugar with no protein or fat.

My point is, the foods you eat, even if they're not sweet, turn into sugar. Keep your blood sugar too high too long and things go out of whack. Think prediabetes and type 2 diabetes. If your blood sugar levels go up and down all the time, you exacerbate anxiety and stress. Anyone with a thyroid condition understands how hard it is to tolerate any kind of stress. If you have thyroid issues, you have to work hard managing your nutrition to make sure your stress doesn't get out of hand. High cortisol (a stress hormone released by the adrenal glands) from chronic stress sets you up for weight gain, particularly around the middle. Cortisol also causes that "tired and wired" feeling, poor sleep, a puffy face, high blood pressure, a weakened immune system, and muscle aches. You know what one of the top causes of stress on the body is? Blood sugar imbalance. Mood swings, cravings, insomnia, and anxiety are signs of imbalanced blood sugar. The solution is balanced eating.

Normal blood sugar is between 80 and 100. When you go to the doctor's office and they do a fasting blood sugar check, that's the range they want to see. That's equal to about one to two teaspoons of sugar in your blood at any given time. If you're not diabetic, your blood sugar should come back down to this range a couple of hours after you eat something. If you have a fasting blood sugar greater than 130 (and blood sugar after a meal greater than 180), you have high blood sugar, also called hyperglycemia.

The standard eating pattern of snacking every few hours ramps up our blood sugar and then drops it again, like an all-day blood sugar roller coaster. This is even worse if you're eating processed junk foods. This roller coaster imbalances and disrupts your blood sugar, eventually causing insulin insensitivity. You might have excessive thirst, blurred vision, brain fog, fatigue, insomnia, depression, or irritability. Ever heard someone joke about being hangry (hungry and angry)? Maybe you've seen those Snickers commercials. They're right about one thing—having symptoms of imbalanced blood sugar puts a lot of stress on the body. I just wouldn't recommend making things worse with a candy bar!

Daily Dose of Cortisol

We're supposed to be awake, thriving, and functioning throughout the day. We're supposed to rest and recover at night. In the morning you're supposed to wake up feeling rested. Remember the stress hormone cortisol? We have four surges of cortisol throughout the day. You have a burst of cortisol in the morning. This gets you ready for your day. Then you have another surge a bit later, when you're at your job or you're doing your thing. This ensures you're still able to focus, concentrate, and have energy to get through your day.

Then afternoon comes, and you have a third cortisol surge. It's a bit lower than that second surge. But again, you should still be thriving and functioning. So many people talk about that afternoon slump, it seems like it's supposed to be normal. But the fact of the matter is, it's not. You should not feel like you need a nap in the afternoon! You shouldn't feel like you can't function for the rest of your day. You shouldn't be falling asleep at your desk or while driving home from work.

Then you have dinner with your family. I know when my kids were little it was always hectic and stressful. Dinner prep, homework, bath time—so much was going on, and I was already tired. I could hardly wait until nighttime.

You have another surge of cortisol at bedtime, and now you're *supposed* to be tired. Ready to go to sleep. You shouldn't be tossing and turning, lying there with your eyes wide and your brain racing. You should come down at night, fall asleep, and then stay asleep until the morning when you have your next cortisol surge.

The problem is this cycle is so out of whack for most of us in our fast-paced American lifestyle. Our cortisol becomes imbalanced, just like our blood sugar. When you have low cortisol, it's because you've been running around all day. It's like running away from a saber-toothed tiger. You trigger your innate fight-or-flight response. Maybe you've felt that response when someone pulled out in front of you on the highway. That adrenaline rush. But when you feel it all the time, when you're always running from the saber-toothed tiger, you burn out. The adrenal glands get tired of helping you function throughout the day. Your high cortisol becomes low cortisol, and you can bounce back and forth between the two.

The good news is, I know with 100 percent certainty that if you get your blood sugar in check, your stress patterns are going to change. That's what simple, balanced meals are going to do for you. Ready to begin?

Week One: Gluten-Free

This week, you have two goals. One is to eat 100 percent gluten-free. The other is to eat balanced macronutrients (carbs, fat, protein) using the meal ideas I give you. I've already told you why eating a gluten-free diet is important to thyroid health, but it also has other benefits—that is, *if* you're eating healthy whole foods rather than relying on gluten-free pretzels and crackers to replace everyday junk food favorites. Some of these gluten-free "replacements" are even more harmful than the gluten. When you replace wheat with high-sugar, low-fiber alternatives, they can actually raise your blood sugar and insulin even more than the wheat! Don't worry. I'll give you tips on how to choose the best alternatives when one is needed.

This week, we're focusing on getting blood sugar imbalance symptoms in check and managing your stress. Including proteins, carbs, and fats every time you eat will decrease stress on the body and help ease the symptoms you may be having. You'll also learn to control cravings, which will make your next steps on this journey far easier.

These meals will be simple. They're not going to be long, drawn-out, scary, weird-ingredient meals, which is part of the point. It's whole food. You know, grab this, grab that, throw it in a pan, mix it together, and boom. We're trying to decrease stress and make your meal prep time efficient so you can get feeling better faster.

First, let's go shopping! You'll be able to buy most things at your regular grocery store. You may need to make a trip to your local health food store or natural food market for a few of these items. As you know, we'll be eliminating dairy next week. If you're used to eating dairy, you can still include it this week. If cheese and sour cream aren't things you already have in the fridge, buy the dairy substitutes I've listed instead. If you're not yet dairy-free, follow the shopping list and meal ideas for Week One as is. Buy everything—dairy and otherwise—organic whenever possible. For meat, buy grass fed, nitrate-free, hormone-free, and antibiotic-free whenever you can.

If you are vegan or vegetarian, there are plant-based protein options you can substitute for the protein sources in the meals listed below. I recommend staying away from gluten- or soy-based vegan proteins such as seitan and tofu. Soy contains a compound called genistein, which some studies suggest may disrupt thyroid hormones. Also, soy is a common food allergen and may contribute to inflammation. I suggest vegetarian protein sources such as chia, lentils, quinoa, chickpeas, and hemp.

One final note on the shopping list and recipe personalization. When I work with people individually, food choices are typically customized or modified depending on their specific health concerns. For most people, the following foods will be perfectly fine. If you have questions about how you may need to adjust any of the upcoming week's meal plans, please reach out to me right away at tiffany@rockbottomwellness.com.

Week One Shopping List

PROTEIN:

- Bacon, 2 ounces
- Beef snack sticks, 2 ounces
- Boneless pork ribs, 4 ounces
- Breakfast sausage, 4 ounces
- Chicken, 32 ounces
- Chicken or steak, 4 ounces (leftover for lunch, Day Five)
- Chicken sausage, 3 ounces
- Eggs, 4
- Ground turkey, 4 ounces
- Hamburger, 4 ounces
- Pork (for pulled pork, dinner, Day Five)
- Protein powder (vanilla or chocolate)
- Sirloin, 4 ounces
- Tuna, canned, wild-caught, 4 ounces
- Turkey slices, 3 ounces

PRODUCE:

- Baby bok choy (regular bok choy is fine, too), 1 head
- Baby spinach, 4 cups
- Bananas, 1 bunch
- Berries, 3 cups (can be a variety)
- Blueberries, 1/2 cup

- Broccoli, 2 cups cooked
- Carrots, 2 large
- Celery, 3 stalks
- Cucumber, 1
- Fresh basil
- Fresh green beans, 2 cups
- Fruit, 1 cup (lunch, Days Six and Seven)
- Grape tomatoes, 2 ounce
- Green bell pepper, 1
- Green onions, 1 bunch
- Greens for salad, 8 cups
- Lettuce, shredded and bagged (for chicken tacos)
- Linguini, gluten-free
- Onion, 1
- Romaine lettuce, 2 cups
- Red bell pepper, 1
- Spaghetti squash, 1
- Tomatoes, 2 small
- Yams, 1
- Yellow bell peppers, 2 large
- Zucchini, 1

DAIRY:

- Butter, 1 teaspoon

- Cheddar cheese, shredded, 3 ounces
- Cottage cheese, 4%, 1 cup
- Cream cheese, 8 ounces, OR Kite Hill brand cream-style "cheese"
- Half-and-half, 2 tablespoon
- Heavy whipping cream, 2 tablespoons
- Milk, 8–12 ounces (or milk substitute like unsweetened almond milk)
- Mozzarella cheese, 3 ounces
- Parmesan cheese
- Ranch dip, 3 tablespoons
- Sour cream, 3 tablespoons (or avocado for Taco Salad)
- Swiss cheese, 1 ounce

FATS/CONDIMENTS/SEASONINGS:

- Almond butter, 1 tablespoon
- Avocado, 1 tablespoon
- Avocado oil
- Black pepper
- Cajun seasoning, gluten-free
- Cayenne
- Cinnamon
- Coconut oil
- Garlic powder
- Chia seeds or flaxseeds, 3 tablespoons

- Flax meal
- Hummus, made with olive oil
- Italian dressing
- Liquid stevia
- Mayonnaise (Mindful Mayo or Just Mayo), 4 tablespoons
- Minced garlic or garlic cloves
- Olive oil
- Pure maple syrup, 1 tablespoon
- Red pepper flakes
- Salsa, 3/4 cup
- Salt
- Smoked paprika
- Sunflower seeds, 2 tablespoons
- Taco seasoning (homemade or Ortega because it's gluten-free)
- Tamari or coconut aminos (coconut aminos are better for thyroid health)
- Toasted sesame oil
- Turmeric
- Vinaigrette dressing

GRAINS/BEANS/SNACKS:

- Black beans, 1/4 cup or 1 can
- Bread, gluten-free, 1–2 loaves
- Corn or black bean tortilla chips

- Crackers, gluten-free (like Nut Thins), 1–2 boxes

- Flour, gluten-free (for pancakes)

- Hamburger buns, gluten-free (or use bread for the burger)

- Jasmine rice, 1/2 cup

- Oatmeal, gluten-free (Glutenfreeda is good)

- Roasted almonds

- Tortillas, gluten-free, 2

- Wild rice, 1/2 cup cooked

Week One Meal Ideas

DAY ONE

BREAKFAST:

2 eggs, cooked any style

Handful baby spinach

2 slices gluten-free toast, 1 tablespoon butter

1/2 cup berries

Total Calories 470

LUNCH:

4-ounce chicken, cooked and diced

2 tablespoons Mindful Mayo or avocado oil

1/2 ounce each diced celery, cucumbers, bell peppers, onion

Smoked paprika, salt, pepper, cayenne, turmeric to taste

1 serving (14 grams) gluten-free crackers (Nut Thins)

Total Calories: 580

DINNER:

4-ounce grilled sirloin

2 cups sautéed green beans and 1/2 cup chopped onions

1–2 tablespoons avocado oil, for cooking

1 teaspoon minced garlic

2½ ounces baked yam, drizzled with 1 teaspoon olive oil and seasoning of your choice

Salt and pepper to taste

Total Calories: 530

SNACKS:

24 roasted almonds

1 small banana

Total Calories: 240

Daily Totals:

Calories: 1,820

Protein: 23% (104 grams)

Carbohydrates: 31% (141 grams)

Fat: 46% (93 grams)

DAY TWO

BREAKFAST:

3 ounces chicken sausage

1/2 cup bell peppers

1/2 cup onions

Cook sausage until almost done, then add veggies and cook in 1 tablespoon avocado or coconut oil until veggies are done to taste.

Total Calories: 260

LUNCH:

> 3 cups spinach salad
>
> 4 ounces grilled chicken
>
> 2 ounces grape tomatoes
>
> 1 ounce mozzarella cheese
>
> 2 tablespoons dressing of choice
>
> 1 serving (14 grams) gluten-free crackers (Nut Thins)

Total Calories: 400

DINNER:

> 4-ounce hamburger patty
>
> 1 tablespoon avocado as burger topping
>
> 2 cups green salad (romaine, spinach, cucumbers, peppers, etc.)
>
> 1 tablespoon dressing of choice
>
> Gluten-free hamburger bun

Total Calories: 590

SNACK:

> Carrot (1/2 cup) and celery (2 stalks) sticks
>
> 2 tablespoons ranch dip

Total Calories: 170

Daily Totals:

> Calories: 1,420
>
> Protein: 21% (74 grams)
>
> Carbohydrates: 37% (131 grams)
>
> Fat: 42% (66 grams)

DAY THREE

BREAKFAST:

1/2 cup gluten-free oatmeal

2 tablespoons half-and-half

Cinnamon to taste

1/2 cup berries

2 ounces breakfast sausage

Total Calories: 285

LUNCH:

Taco Salad

4 ounces taco meat (ground turkey)

2 cups romaine lettuce

1/4 cup salsa

1/4 cup black beans

1 tablespoon sour cream or avocado

1 ounce shredded cheddar cheese

1 serving corn or black bean tortilla chips

Total Calories: 500

DINNER:

4 ounces boneless pork ribs, seasoned to taste

1/2 cup wild rice, cooked

2 cups steamed broccoli

1 tablespoon olive oil drizzled over broccoli and seasoned with salt and pepper to taste

Total Calories: 510

SNACK:

  2 ounces beef snack sticks

  1/2 cucumber, sliced

  1 tablespoon ranch dip

Total Calories: 260

Daily Totals

  Calories: 1,555

  Protein: 26% (104 grams)

  Carbohydrates: 27% (106 grams)

  Fat: 47% (81 grams)

DAY FOUR

BREAKFAST:

  Protein Smoothie

  1 scoop protein powder

  4–8 ounces milk or milk substitute

  1 tablespoon flaxseeds or chia seeds

  1/3 banana

  2 sausage links or 1 sausage patty

Total Calories: 355

LUNCH:

  4 ounces canned tuna

  2 tablespoon mayonnaise

  1½ stalks celery

  2 cups salad greens

  1 tablespoon sunflower seeds

  1 tablespoon dressing of choice

  1 serving gluten-free crackers

Total Calories: 525

DINNER:

Chicken Taco

4-ounce chicken breast, shredded, seasoned with taco seasoning

1/4 cup salsa

Shredded lettuce

1 ounce shredded cheddar cheese

1–2 tablespoons sour cream

1–2 gluten-free tortillas, warmed

Total Calories: 565

SNACK:

1 cup berries

2 tablespoons whipped heavy cream

1 drop liquid stevia (if desired)

1 tablespoon sunflower seeds

Total Calories: 150

Daily Totals:

Calories: 1,595

Protein: 25% (101 grams)

Carbohydrates: 28% (113 grams)

Fat: 47% (83 grams)

DAY FIVE

BREAKFAST:

1 cup 4% cottage cheese

1/2 cup blueberries

1 tablespoon flax meal, flaxseeds, or chia seeds

1 slice gluten-free toast, 1 teaspoon butter

Total Calories: 470

LUNCH:

4 ounces leftover steak, chicken, or pork

2–3 cups salad greens

Other veggies you desire

Ranch dressing

1 slice gluten-free toast, 1 teaspoon butter

Total Calories: 315

DINNER:

4 ounces pulled pork

1 gluten-free bun/bread OR eat pork alone

Salad with 1 tablespoon dressing of choice

Total Calories: 390

SNACK:

Mini Smoothie

1/2 scoop protein powder

4 ounces milk or milk substitute

1/2 tablespoon olive oil

1/2 cup berries

Total Calories: 155

Daily Totals:

Calories: 1,330

Protein: 26% (86 grams)

Carbohydrates: 42% (141 grams)

Fat: 32% (48 grams)

DAY SIX

BREAKFAST:

3 pancakes, made with gluten-free flour substitute, cooked in almond butter

1 tablespoon almond butter

1/2–1 tablespoon pure maple syrup

1/4 cup berries

Total Calories: 380

LUNCH:

Chef salad with 2 tablespoons dressing of choice

1 slice gluten-free toast, 1 teaspoon butter

1/2 cup fruit

Total Calories: 580

DINNER:

Creamy Cajun Chicken Pasta (recipe below)

Cooked zoodles (a zucchini shredded into noodles with a potato peeler or a spiralizer, or you can buy them precut)

4 boneless chicken breasts, cut into strips

1 bunch green onions, sliced

1 green pepper, diced

1 red pepper, cut into strips

2 tablespoons Cajun seasoning (less or more depending on how hot you like your food)

1 teaspoon garlic powder

1 8-ounce container Kite Hill cream-style "cheese"

2 ounces unsweetened coconut milk or almond milk

2 tablespoons coconut oil

Salt and pepper to taste

Creamy Cajun Chicken Pasta Directions

Slice chicken into strips and season with Cajun spices. Set aside and cut up the veggies. Heat pan to medium-high and add coconut oil. Cook chicken until tender. Drain extra liquid. Add peppers and other seasonings to pan and cook until peppers are tender but slightly crispy. Once peppers are done, lower heat and add heavy cream and green onion. Serve over 1/2 cup gluten-free linguini or spaghetti squash, or eat it plain like I do.

Options:

● Add mushrooms (with green onions), broccoli (with peppers), or any other veggie you like.

● Add parmesan cheese or nutritional yeast for cheesier topping.

Total Calories: 350

SNACK:

2 ounces mozzarella cheese

1 small tomato

Baby spinach leaves

2 tablespoons vinaigrette dressing

Fresh basil

Total Calories: 320

Daily Totals:

Calories: 1,630

Protein: 16% (65 grams)

Carbohydrates: 28% (115 grams)

Fat: 56% (102 grams)

DAY SEVEN

BREAKFAST:

2 eggs, cooked in grape seed oil

1/4 cup chopped onion

1 ounce shredded cheddar cheese

2 ounces nitrate-free bacon or sausage

1 slice gluten-free toast, 1 teaspoon butter

Total Calories: 410

LUNCH:

Turkey and Swiss Sandwich

2 slices gluten-free bread

3 ounces turkey slices

1 ounce swiss cheese

3 tomato slices

1 lettuce leaf (or as much as the sandwich can hold)

1 tablespoon dressing of choice or mayo

1/2 cup fruit

Total Calories: 500

DINNER:

Bok Choy Chicken Stir-Fry (recipe below)

1 tablespoon coconut oil

1 tablespoon toasted sesame oil

1 chicken breast, cut into pieces

2 large yellow bell peppers, sliced

1 onion, chopped

1 baby bok choy, chopped

Tamari, soy sauce, or coconut aminos

Red pepper flakes to taste

Salt and pepper to taste

1/2 cup jasmine rice

Bok Choy Chicken Stir-Fry Directions

Heat coconut oil in a large sauté pan on high heat. Add chicken and stir-fry until lightly browned. Remove and set aside. Add sesame oil to pan and stir-fry onion and peppers until lightly browned. Add chicken to vegetable mixture, lower the heat to medium, add bok choy, and toss until wilted. The thicker ends will be somewhat crunchy. While bok choy is cooking, add tamari, coconut aminos, or soy sauce to taste along with red pepper flakes, salt, and pepper. Serve with jasmine rice.

Total Calories: 586

SNACK:

1 serving (14 grams) gluten-free crackers (Nut Thins)

2 tablespoons hummus

Total Calories: 200

Daily Totals:

Calories: 1,696

Protein: 20% (81 grams)

Carbohydrates: 46% (190 grams)

Fat: 34% (63 grams)

Week Two: Gluten- and Dairy-Free

Congratulations! You've completed Week One of the Rock Bottom Thyroid Reset. You're working on transitioning from gluten to non gluten grains while cleaning up your diet. This week, you're going to continue eating balanced macronutrients—protein, carbs, fat— while remaining gluten-free. You now have an additional goal— add (or take away, rather) dairy.

The issue with dairy can be twofold. Some people have an intolerance to the sugar in dairy (lactose). It can cause major digestive upset—no fun at all! It can be painful and embarrassing.

Like gluten, dairy causes inflammation, especially for people with thyroid issues. If you're already lactose intolerant, your body doesn't produce the enzyme lactase to break down lactose (again, sugar in dairy). But lactose isn't the only problem. Casein and whey (protein in dairy) can be bad news for people with thyroid issues. Gluten-sensitive people are often sensitive to whey and casein as well. Bottom line—dairy is difficult for the body to digest. That's why it's important to go dairy-free while you're improving your thyroid health.

Dairy-sensitive people often clear their throat, feel stuffy, have a runny nose, and may even feel some swelling in their hands, feet, and joints after eating dairy. Often people are so used to consuming dairy throughout the day, they're not even aware they have these symptoms. It takes a spouse who's annoyed with throat clearing to point out the improvement. Taking these inflammatory culprits out of the diet can help you realize how you've been reacting to them in the first place.

As you do your shopping for this week, read those ingredient labels. You'll find casein in prepackaged deli meats as a filler or binder and in other products like coffee creamers labeled as non dairy. The thing is, if you're buying whole foods, you usually don't even see a label. Fruits, veggies, beans, nuts, seeds, grains (other than wheat, barley, and oats), meat, and eggs are all naturally gluten- and dairy-free.

Follow the Week Two meal ideas or use them as guidelines. Remember, the idea is to get a complete meal—protein, carbohydrates, and fat—to balance your blood sugar and keep cravings at bay.

Speaking of blood sugar, we're going to give your body extra rest this week. Caffeinated beverages, sodas, and artificially sweetened beverages are hard on your liver. To avoid unpleasant side effects from quitting these cold turkey, cut back gradually. Make it your goal to eliminate them entirely by the end of the week. If you think you can handle the side effects (headaches and moodiness), stop drinking these beverages now. Instead drink plenty of water—plain, sparkling, or flavored sparkling. You can buy stevia liquid drops to flavor your water. I also enjoy decaffeinated or herbal (naturally caffeine-free) tea.

Week Two Shopping List

PROTEIN:

- Bacon, 2 ounces
- Beef snack sticks, 2 ounces
- Boneless pork ribs, 4 ounces
- Breakfast sausage, 4 ounces
- Chicken, 12 ounces
- Chicken sausage, 3 ounces
- Eggs, 6
- Flank steak, 4 ounces
- Ground sausage, 2 ounces
- Ground turkey, 8 ounces
- Protein powder (vanilla or chocolate)

- Rotisserie chicken, 7 ounces
- Sausage links, 2, or sausage patty, 1
- Tuna, canned, wild-caught, 4 ounces
- Turkey slices, 3 ounces

DAIRY ALTERNATIVES:

- Coconut milk, 1 can (not lite)
- Kite Hill cream-style "cheese"
- Unsweetened almond or coconut milk, 1 carton

FATS/CONDIMENTS/SEASONINGS:

- Almond butter
- Avocado oil
- Avocado, 1
- Black pepper
- Chia seeds or flaxseeds, 2 tablespoons
- Coconut aminos
- Coconut oil
- Garlic salt
- Green Goddess Dressing by Primal Kitchen
- Guacamole, 2 tablespoons, or Wholly Guacamole Mini cups
- Hummus, made with olive oil
- Mindful Mayo or Just Mayo, 2 tablespoons
- Olive oil
- Pumpkin or sunflower seeds, 1 tablespoon
- Pure maple syrup, 1 tablespoon
- Salad Girl dressing
- Salsa, 1/2 cup

- Salt
- Sliced almonds, 1 ounce
- Spaghetti sauce, 1/2 cups
- Sunflower seeds, 3 tablespoons

GRAINS/BEANS/SNACKS:

- Black beans, 1/4 cup or 1 can
- Bread, gluten-free, 1–2 loaves
- Corn or black bean tortilla chips
- Crackers, gluten-free (like Nut Thins), 1–2 boxes
- Flour, gluten-free (for pancakes)
- Oatmeal, gluten-free (Glutenfreeda is good)
- Quinoa, 3/4 cup cooked
- Roasted almonds, 2 servings

Week Two Meal Ideas

DAY ONE

BREAKFAST:

    2 eggs, cooked any style

    1/2 cup diced bell pepper and onion

    1 teaspoon avocado oil, for cooking

    1 slice gluten-free toast, 1/2 teaspoon almond butter

    1/2 cup berries

Total Calories 430

Carbohydrates: 37 grams

Protein: 20 grams

Fat: 23 grams

LUNCH:

Protein Bowl

2 cups lettuce or mixed greens

4 ounces rotisserie chicken

1/4 cup cooked quinoa

1/2 tablespoon pumpkin or sunflower seeds

1/4 cup diced apples

2 tablespoons Salad Girl dressing

Combine salad and quinoa, add dressing and coat evenly, add the remaining ingredients.

1 serving (14 grams) gluten-free crackers (Nut Thins)

Total Calories: 470

Carbohydrates: 54 grams

Protein: 21 grams

Fat: 13 grams

DINNER:

4 ounces grilled chicken, cut into strips

1 cup spaghetti squash, cooked (see below)

1/2 tablespoon olive oil, drizzled on squash

Garlic salt and pepper to taste

1 cup bagged, chopped salad (like Taylor Farms)

1–2 tablespoons dairy-free dressing of choice

To prepare spaghetti squash, cut squash lengthwise, remove seeds, and place facedown in a bit of water in bottom of baking dish. Bake in oven at 350°F for about 30 minutes, depending on size. Using a fork, shred cooked squash into spaghetti-like strands.

Total Calories: 470

Carbohydrates: 27 grams

Protein: 28 grams

Fat: 27 grams

SNACKS:

Roasted almonds (45 grams)

1/2 medium banana

Total Calories: 270

Carbohydrate: 22 grams

Protein: 9 grams

Fat: 24 grams

Daily Totals:

Calories: 1,640

Protein: 19% (78 grams)

Carbohydrates: 34% (140 grams)

Fat: 47% (87 grams)

DAY TWO

BREAKFAST:

> 3 ounces chicken sausage
>
> 1/2 cup bell peppers
>
> 1/2 cup onions
>
> Cook sausage until almost done, then add veggies and cook in 1 teaspoon avocado or coconut oil until veggies are done to taste.

Total Calories: 200

Carbohydrates: 16 grams

Protein: 15 grams

Fat: 9 grams

LUNCH:

> 4 ounces grilled chicken
>
> 3 cups baby spinach
>
> 1 ounce sliced cucumbers
>
> 1 ounce bell peppers, chopped
>
> 1 tablespoon sunflower seeds
>
> 2 tablespoons dairy-free dressing of choice
>
> 1 serving (14 grams) gluten-free crackers (Nut Thins)

Total Calories: 630

Carbohydrates: 39 grams

Protein: 57 grams

Fat: 22 grams

DINNER:

Paleo Smoothie

1 scoop PurePaleo protein powder

1 tablespoon almond butter

1/2 medium banana

8 ounces unsweetened almond milk

Add any greens you like to boost the nutrition.

Total Calories: 280

Carbohydrates: 20 grams

Protein: 13 grams

Fat: 26 grams

SNACK:

Carrot (1/2 cup) and celery (2 stalks) sticks

2 tablespoons hummus

Total Calories: 130

Carbohydrates: 16 grams

Protein: 2 grams

Fat: 5 grams

Daily Totals:

Calories: 1,240

Protein: 27% (87 grams)

Carbohydrates: 28% (91 grams)

Fat: 45% (62 grams)

DAY THREE

BREAKFAST:

1/2 cup gluten-free oatmeal

1/4 cup almond or coconut milk

Cinnamon to taste

1/2 cup berries

2 ounces breakfast sausage

Total Calories: 285

Carbohydrates: 37 grams

Protein: 15 grams

Fat: 18 grams

LUNCH:

Taco Salad

4 ounces taco meat (ground turkey)

2 cups romaine lettuce

1/4–1/2 cup salsa

1/4 cup black beans

1–2 tablespoons guacamole or Wholly Guacamole Mini cup

1 serving corn or black bean tortilla chips

Total Calories: 465

Carbohydrates: 37 grams

Protein: 29 grams

Fat: 24 grams

DINNER:

4 ounces boneless pork ribs, seasoned to taste

3 ounces baked sweet potato

2 cups steamed broccoli

1 tablespoon olive oil drizzled over broccoli and seasoned with salt and pepper to taste

Total Calories: 530

Carbohydrates: 35 grams

Protein: 42 grams

Fat: 25 grams

SNACK:

2 ounces beef snack sticks

1/2 cup cucumber slices

2 tablespoons hummus

Total Calories: 275

Carbohydrates: 4 grams

Protein: 12 grams

Fat: 23 grams

Daily Totals:

Calories: 1,555

Protein: 23% (98 grams)

Carbohydrates: 27% (113 grams)

Fat: 50% (90 grams)

DAY FOUR

BREAKFAST:

Protein Smoothie

1 scoop protein powder (vanilla or chocolate)

4–8 ounces milk substitute

1 tablespoon flaxseeds or chia seeds

1/3 banana

2 sausage links or 1 sausage patty

Total Calories: 325

Carbohydrates: 17 grams

Protein: 31 grams

Fat: 15 grams

LUNCH:

4 ounces canned tuna

2 tablespoons mayonnaise

1½ stalks celery

2 cups salad greens

1 tablespoon sunflower seeds

1 serving (14 grams) gluten-free crackers (Nut Thins)

Total Calories: 510

Carbohydrates: 30 grams

Protein: 27 grams

Fat: 29 grams

DINNER:

    4-ounce flank steak

    1/2 cup quinoa, cooked

    1 ounce onions and peppers

    2 cups chopped salad

    1–2 tablespoons dairy-free dressing of choice

Total Calories: 560

Carbohydrates: 59 grams

Protein: 35 grams

Fat: 14 grams

SNACK:

    1 cup berries

    2 tablespoons whipped coconut cream

    1 drop liquid stevia (if desired)

    1 tablespoon sunflower seeds

Total Calories: 300

Carbohydrates: 22 grams

Protein: 6 grams

Fat: 20 grams

Daily Totals:

    Calories: 1,695

    Protein: 26% (99 grams)

    Carbohydrates: 32% (125 grams)

    Fat: 45% (78 grams)

DAY FIVE

BREAKFAST:

2 slices gluten-free toast

2 tablespoons olive oil

Garlic salt, pepper, or other seasoning to taste

1/2 avocado, sliced

1 tablespoon flax meal, flaxseeds, or chia seeds

Top toast with olive oil and seasonings, add avocado slices, and sprinkle with chia seeds or flaxseeds.

Total Calories: 560

Carbohydrates: 32 grams

Protein: 7 grams

Fat: 46 grams

LUNCH:

4 ounces leftover steak, chicken, or pork

2–3 cups salad greens

Other veggies you desire

1 tablespoon dairy-free dressing of choice

1 slice gluten-free toasted bread, made into garlic toast with avocado oil and garlic salt

Total Calories: 540

Carbohydrates: 33 grams

Protein: 38 grams

Fat: 27 grams

DINNER:

  4 ounces pulled pork

  1 gluten-free bun/bread OR eat pork alone

  3 cups salad greens

  1 tablespoon dairy-free dressing of choice

Total Calories: 488

Carbohydrates: 71 grams

Protein: 21 grams

Fat: 13 grams

SNACK:

  Mini Smoothie

  1/2 scoop protein powder (vanilla or chocolate)

  4 ounces milk substitute

  1/2 tablespoon olive oil

  1/2 cup berries

Total Calories: 170

Carbohydrates: 12 grams

Protein: 11 grams

Fat: 9 grams

Daily Totals:

  Calories: 1,758

  Protein: 20% (94 grams)

  Carbohydrates: 32% (148 grams)

  Fat: 48% (95 grams)

DAY SIX

BREAKFAST:

3 pancakes, made with gluten-free flour substitute, cooked in coconut oil

1 tablespoon almond butter

1/2–1 tablespoon pure maple syrup

1/4 cup berries

Total Calories: 409

Carbohydrates: 62 grams

Protein: 8 grams

Fat: 13 grams

LUNCH:

Green Goddess Cobb Salad

3 cups salad greens

3 ounces rotisserie chicken

1 roma tomato, quartered

1/4 cup red onion, sliced

1 hard-boiled egg

1/4 cup chopped bacon

1/2 avocado, sliced

1 tablespoon Green Goddess Dressing by Primal Kitchen

Total Calories: 620

Carbohydrates: 20 grams

Protein: 37 grams

Fat: 41 grams

DINNER:

    6 ounces zoodles

    1/2 cup spaghetti sauce

    4 ounces ground turkey

    1 cup steamed broccoli

Total Calories: 422

Carbohydrates: 30 grams

Protein: 29 grams

Fat: 22 grams

SNACK:

    1 cup berries

    1/4 cup whipped coconut cream (whipped from canned coconut milk after draining off liquid)

    24 almonds

Total Calories: 360

Carbohydrates: 22 grams

Protein: 7 grams

Fat: 31 grams

Daily Totals:

    Calories: 1,811

    Protein: 18% (81 grams)

    Carbohydrates: 29% (134 grams)

    Fat: 53% (107 grams)

DAY SEVEN

BREAKFAST:

Egg Scramble:

3 eggs

1/4 cup chopped onion

1/4 cup chopped bell peppers

1/4 cup chopped mushrooms

2 ounces ground sausage

Whisk eggs and add remainder of ingredients. Cook with 1 tablespoon avocado or coconut oil.

1/2 medium banana or other fruit

Total Calories: 600

Carbohydrates: 23 grams

Protein: 32 grams

Fat: 41 grams

LUNCH:

Herb Turkey Sandwich

2 slices gluten-free bread

3 turkey slices

2 tablespoons Kite Hill cream-style "cheese"

3 tomato slices

1 lettuce leaf (or as much as the sandwich can hold)

1 medium apple

Total Calories: 400

Carbohydrates: 53 grams

Protein: 17 grams

Fat: 13 grams

DINNER:

    4-ounce grilled chicken breast, seasoned to taste

    1/2 cup baked sweet potato

    1 cup sautéed green beans

    2 tablespoons coconut aminos (for sautéing green beans)

    1 ounce sliced almonds (sautéed with beans)

    1 tablespoon avocado or coconut oil

Total Calories: 440

Carbohydrates: 38 grams

Protein: 33 grams

Fat: 30 grams

SNACK:

    1 serving (14 grams) gluten-free crackers (Nut Thins)

    2 tablespoons hummus

Total Calories: 200

Carbohydrates: 27 grams

Protein: 5 grams

Fat: 7 grams

Daily Totals

    Calories: 1,640

    Protein: 20% (91 grams)

    Carbohydrates: 32% (141 grams)

    Fat: 48% (63 grams)

R

CHAPTER 5

Rock Bottom Thyroid Reset: Phase Two

"My life has completely changed. I have managed to cut out gluten and all bread, of course. No beer, cookies, cakes, or donuts. I won't lie, that part was hard. But after trial and error, I now know I do have a gluten sensitivity without a doubt. I am off the sleeping pills—yippie! And my biggest accomplishment so far, I just completed a six-week New You Challenge at Una Stamus Fitness in Elk River."

— Henry C., Elk River, Minnesota

The Detox Phase: Give Your Liver a Break

We've all heard of detoxification. You'll hear someone make light of detoxing when a friend has too many drinks. But detoxification is not a one-off diet. Detox is a constant process the liver is involved in (along with our skin, kidneys, and lungs) to keep us healthy. Detoxification is simply the body getting rid of "junk" every second of every day. It has to! We live in an increasingly toxic civilization. These toxins remain in our environment for years. We have to combat these toxins *and* the chemical-laden foods we've eaten for years.

Toxins can and do get trapped in our organs and tissues, wearing down our bodies over time. Liver to the rescue! The liver detoxifies our bodies from all these harmful substances we eat, breathe in, and absorb through our skin.

But I already eat healthy. I don't smoke or drink. Do I still need to detox?

Detoxification is not just about what you eat. Let me show you what we're bombarded with daily. Each and every second, industrial facilities around the world release 310 kilograms of toxic chemicals into our air, water, and land. Many are carcinogens, known cancer-causing agents. And that stat doesn't cover the chemicals in the foods we eat every day! You can't go a day without hearing of someone newly diagnosed with cancer or in the fight of their life against it. Toxins deserve a large part of the blame.

I don't say this to scare you. I say this to show you how important it is to support the body's natural detox process. Thank goodness our bodies strive to keep us healthy, repair damage, and maintain balance. So how can you help your liver do its thing?

In Weeks Three and Four of the Rock Bottom Thyroid Reset, I'm going to show you how to give your liver the support it needs to function at its optimal level. Your meals and beverages will supercharge the detox process. How? You're basically going to give your liver a rest by eliminating even more junk foods and unhealthy beverages. That's not all. Our liver needs specific nutrients to get us through the first step of detoxification. These nutrients include B vitamins like folate, minerals like calcium, amino acids like NAC (N-acetyl cysteine), herbs like milk thistle, and bioflavonoids like quercetin. In this first step, your liver will convert toxins like microorganisms, pollutants, pesticides, food additives, drugs, and even alcohol into less harmful substances.

In the second step of detoxification, your liver will add other substances to the now-neutralized toxins so your body can release them via bile, urine, or feces. To do this, your body needs amino acids from quality protein, cruciferous vegetables, and calcium d-glucarate to name a few. As you can see, detox is a methodical process. Don't worry: you're not in this alone, and you don't have to figure out how to get these nutrients. I'm going to give you all the tools you need to support your liver and rid your body of toxins in the way it does best.

Frequently Asked Detox Questions

Here are the types of questions I often hear from my clients when they begin the Rock Bottom Thyroid Reset.

"Will the detox be uncomfortable?"

Everybody has a different response to dietary changes. Your transition into the detox should feel easy since you've prepped your body. After all, you've closely followed my recommendations for the last two weeks. The Detox Phase is *not* a fast or a colon cleanse—both of which can be hard on your system. You'll eat plenty of food (and it's delicious!). During the first few days, you may have withdrawal symptoms from sugar and caffeine like mild headache or fatigue. This will vary depending on how well you followed phase one of the reset. If you do feel withdrawal, it will pass. Be patient. It'll be worth it!

"So the detox could give me headaches?"

Some people experience mild headaches during the first few days of the Rock Bottom Thyroid Reset due to sugar and caffeine withdrawal. Because most of my clients prepare themselves well during phase one, they don't have to worry about migraines. I've carefully chosen the protein I'll have you eat over the next two weeks to help your body process sugar and caffeine withdrawal as fast as possible.

"Will I be in the bathroom all day?"

No, the Detox Phase is not a harsh cleanse or a colon cleanse. It is, however, important to consume plenty of water while detoxing to help flush out toxins. So most people urinate more often than usual, but not "all day."

"Will the detox help me lose weight?"

Neither the detox nor the other phases are weight-loss programs. Weight loss is an outcome, an effect, a benefit of detoxing your body and eating whole foods. That's why so many people lose weight during the Detox Phase. You're removing inflammatory foods and eating fewer calories. You're also reducing the sugar in your diet, releasing toxins from fat stores, and leaving common allergenic foods off your plate. Releasing weight by releasing this inflammation shouldn't be minimized as just "water weight." This weight loss helps your body heal and start feeling really well in a short time.

"Can I exercise during the detox?"

If you're feeling up to it, by all means exercise. Monitor yourself, of course. On days you feel fatigued, limit yourself to gentle movement such as stretching, walking, or yoga. Although I do recommend light to moderate exercise, I don't think it's a good idea to take on high-intensity exercise or start a new program during your detox.

"What if I take vitamins and supplements? Should I stop during the detox?"

The protein shakes you'll be drinking over the next two weeks contain vitamins and nutrients that help you meet your daily needs. If you wish, you may stop taking other supplements during this phase under the guidance of your health care practitioner. Continue to take any medically prescribed pharmaceuticals.

"So I'm not allowed to eat anything but kale, right?"

Not quite. Vegetables are good for you, but eating nothing but veggies can do more harm than good! Ever heard of a fruit and veggie fast? If so, you've probably also heard how difficult they are. Weakness is a common complaint. That's not due to the lack of calories. You get a lot of vitamins and minerals from fruits and vegetables but usually not enough protein and other nutrients your liver needs to detox your body. Fruit and vegetable fasts can be ok for a couple of days but to truly support the liver, you need more than that.

The Rock Bottom Thyroid Reset is different. Your meal plans for the day support your body's detoxification process. Even when you're not actively detoxing, you can still help the natural process along by staying away from unnecessary chemicals and toxins. All you have to do is choose high-quality foods. Let me show you how.

General Rock Bottom Thyroid Reset Guidelines

Eat whole foods that are in season if possible. Shop the perimeter of the grocery store where fresh whole foods are usually displayed, and try to avoid (or eliminate) things resembling a "healthier" version of the foods you would normally eat. The only exception might be zoodles instead of spaghetti—zucchini is a whole food! Avoid overly processed and packaged foods whenever possible.

Eliminate sugars, desserts, and artificial sweeteners. Feel free to include natural, low-impact sweeteners such as stevia, monk fruit, and sugar alcohols such as erythritol or xylitol. These are *not* artificial sweeteners (like aspartame, saccharin, and sucralose). Sugar alcohols cause GI discomfort in some people, but most people tolerate them well in moderation. Pay attention to how you feel. (Caution: xylitol can be dangerous to dogs and cats!)

Continue your gluten-free eating over the next two weeks. That means no pastas, bread, crackers, cereals, and other products that contain wheat, oats, rye, spelt, kamut, bulgur, couscous, or barley. Leave dairy products like milk, cheese, ice cream, and yogurt out of your diet as well. Gluten-free whole grains such as brown rice, wild rice, millet, quinoa, amaranth, and buckwheat are okay in moderation. I emphasize—*in moderation.* Gluten-free grains and flours spike blood sugar. It's easy to overuse them. If you want to give gluten-free grain alternatives a try, eat no more than a quarter to a half cup each day. Some may not be able to tolerate even that amount depending on your specific health status and goals.

For protein, I recommend lean, clean, quality choices such as organic grass-fed meat, eggs, and poultry. Avoid pork and pork products. Wild cold-water fish is better than farm-raised, but avoid fish known to be high in mercury such as swordfish, shark, tuna steak, king mackerel, halibut, and tilefish. Good sources of vegetarian or vegan proteins include beans, quinoa, hemp, hummus (chickpeas), and almond, cashew, and sunflower seed butter.

Weight Loss and Detox Suggestions

Want to boost your weight loss during the detox? Then I have a few modifications you can make to your diet and lifestyle over the next two weeks. That said, everybody is different, and every *body* responds to different foods in different ways. You can try all of these suggestions or none. If you do remove the foods and beverages listed below, add them back to your diet at the end of the detox one at a time. This way, you'll be able to tell which work for your body and which cause symptoms. Let's start with drinks.

Alcoholic beverages, caffeinated beverages, sodas, and artificially sweetened beverages give your liver a hard time. I suggest you eliminate them for this detox. I advise most clients to continue to be free of them in the future. Instead of coffee, sodas, and artificially sweetened beverages, drink plain or sparkling water, preferably purified. You can buy flavored liquid stevia drops to flavor your water. You can also enjoy decaffeinated or herbal tea. As a rule of thumb, drink a half ounce of water per pound of body weight every day during this detox. For example, a two-hundred-pound person should drink one hundred ounces of water a day.

To help boost weight loss, you can try drinking one cup of hot water with a quarter of a lemon squeezed into it and two pinches of cayenne pepper first thing in the morning (on an empty stomach). It sounds simple, but you'd be amazed how many people say they can't live without it once they start. Lemon cayenne water supports your liver, boosts your immune system, and helps with weight loss. Take a warm bath with a cup of Epsom salts added to soothe, relax, and further detox your body. Rub on the salt with a warm, wet washcloth in the bath or shower. Invigorating! And prepare your own hydrotherapy in the shower by alternating hot and cold water. This stimulates the circulation and your immune system. If you belong to a gym, alternate between the sauna and a cold shower. Try five to ten minutes of each repeated twice.

Tune in to your body and make sure that you're truly hungry—not bored, tired, or stressed—when you eat. Instead of raiding the refrigerator for comfort food, try lemon cayenne water, warm Epsom salt baths, or hydrotherapy.

To enhance your detox, limit beans in your meals. Beans are a source of protein and carbohydrates—too many carbs for people who have blood sugar instability or those who have trouble losing weight. The lectins in beans can be bothersome to people so preparing (soaking before cooking) them right is essential if you're one of those people. Avoid them altogether or limit your serving size to half a cup a couple of times per week. No more.

Fruits naturally contain nutrients and antioxidants as well as fiber. Depending on how your body feels and functions with certain foods, you may need to moderate fruit for a bit. One reason to limit them is fructose (i.e., fruit sugar), which impacts your liver and therefore your blood sugar levels (the liver metabolizes fructose). If you don't want to avoid all fruit, blend berries in your morning shake. Berries have a lower glycemic index than apples or pears, for example. If you've ever found it hard to lose weight, leaving all moderate- to high-glycemic fruits out of your diet (and your drinks) for the next two weeks will be helpful.

Like beans and fruits, nuts and seeds are healthy but can sabotage your weight-loss efforts. Even though they're full of good fats and protein, it may be too high in carbohydrates for some. In addition, it is often hard to moderate the amount of nuts and seeds we eat when we grab them by the handful. If weight loss isn't a priority, eat only a half ounce (two tablespoons) of nuts and seeds once or twice a day.

When you're making your protein shakes, you can drizzle in olive oil or one serving of nut butter of your choice to increase satiety and to avoid the blood sugar drop that causes cravings. If you're avoiding nuts, you could add chia seeds or flax meal for the same purpose.

Suggestions aside, I want you to remember that the Rock Bottom Thyroid Reset is not a calorie-restrictive program. If you feel hungry between meals, snack on healthy whole foods in moderation. I've provided you with a list of delicious snack options below.

The Rock Bottom Thyroid Reset, Phase Two: Simple Schedule

Consume two protein shakes (recipe below) per day and one healthy meal. This shake mix is professional grade and meets the highest level of testing for quality and efficacy. Protein shakes are designed to help all phases of detoxification. They have a robust nutrient profile. You may consume these shakes and healthy meals at convenient times in your daily schedule. You may also snack on healthy whole foods in moderation.

To make your protein shake:

In a blender, mix one serving (2 scoops) shake mix in water or your choice of unsweetened almond milk, coconut milk, or other milk alternative. Add one of the healthy fat options to increase satiety. And add a few berries if you wish.

Healthy Food and Snack Options

CLEAN PROTEIN OPTIONS

● Bison

● Cold-water fish (salmon, cod, sardines, Pacific flounder/sole, butterfish, and trout—choose wild ocean fish over farm-raised fish)

● Grass-fed beef

● Lamb

● Nitrate-free turkey

● Organic eggs

● Organic legumes (acceptable as a vegetarian protein)

● Organic/hormone-free chicken

OPTIMAL FAT CHOICES

● Avocado

● Coconut oil

● Extra-virgin olive oil

● Flaxseed

● Hemp seed

● Raw, sprouted, or dry-roasted nuts and seeds

● Walnut oil

LOW-GLYCEMIC FRUITS

● Berries (blueberries, strawberries, raspberries, blackberries, etc.)

MODERATE-GLYCEMIC FRUITS (fresh or frozen—limit to a few times per week or avoid)

- Apples
- Apricots
- Cherries
- Grapefruit
- Kiwi
- Melons (not watermelon)
- Nectarines
- Oranges
- Peaches
- Pears
- Plums
- Tangerines

BEVERAGES

- Herbal tea
- Naturally decaffeinated green tea
- Plain or sparkling purified water

VEGETABLE CHOICES

You can eat an unlimited amount of vegetables from the list below. Limit or avoid starchy veggies such as potatoes and sweet potatoes.

- Bell peppers
- Bok choy

- Carrots

- Cruciferous vegetables (kale, brussels sprouts, cabbage, cauliflower, broccoli)

- Cucumbers

- Portabella mushrooms

- Raw sauerkraut (in the refrigerated section—if it's on the shelf, it's not raw)

- Salad greens (lettuce, spinach, etc.)

CONDIMENTS

- Capers

- Cayenne pepper

- Cilantro

- Cumin

- Flax/olive oil and raw apple cider vinegar for dressings

- Fresh herbs and spices

- Garlic

- Garlic pesto

- Lemon

- Lime

- Sea salt

- Tomato pesto

MISCELLANEOUS SNACK OPTIONS

- Bone broth

- Hummus (made with olive oil)

- Low-glycemic fruit
- Nuts and nut butters (raw is best)
- Raw or steamed veggies
- Veggie soup
- Veggie broth

Snack Examples:

Almond butter and apple slices and/or celery sticks

1 piece of fruit and 10 to 12 almonds, walnuts, or pecans

Cut-up carrots or bell peppers with 1–2 tablespoons of hummus

Turkey roll-up: Place chopped tomato, cucumber, 1/4 avocado, and grated carrot in the middle of a slice of nitrate-free turkey. Roll turkey around the veggies and avocado. Add salsa or hummus for variety.

Sample Breakfast Menus

Use these quick meals when you prefer to have your two shakes for lunch and dinner.

2–3 hard-boiled eggs with 1/2 grapefruit

2/3 cup hot quinoa cereal or gluten-free steel-cut oats, 1/2–1 scoop of protein powder, 1/2 cup berries, and a small handful of walnuts or pecans

Detox Scramble: 2–3 eggs, scrambled with onion and/or garlic and broccoli

Add leftover protein from the night before to sautéed veggies, stir to heat up, and season to taste with spices

2–3 poached eggs over a bed of fresh spinach and sliced tomato

2–3 slices turkey bacon with sliced tomato and avocado

Sample Lunch and Dinner Menus

Use these when you prefer to have your two shakes for breakfast and either lunch or dinner.

Green salad with sprouts, extra-virgin olive oil, basil, and squeezed lemon or lime

Mixed green or baby greens salad with extra-virgin olive oil and squeezed lemon or lime

Baked fish or chicken topped with avocado salsa: chop and combine 1 avocado, 1 tomato, and 1/2 cup red onion; add 1/2 cup capers (drained), 1/4 cup fresh cilantro, 1/2 teaspoon cumin, 1/4 teaspoon cayenne, and 2 tablespoons lime juice

1 cup spicy tomatoes and black beans

Chopped cabbage with chicken and apple cider vinegar

Chicken (or shrimp) and vegetables: sauté fresh chicken/shrimp and chopped garlic in a pan with coconut oil over medium heat; roughly chop 5–10 different vegetables and lightly stir-fry with freshly grated ginger and 1/2 cup zucchini noodles until heated through; lightly drizzle with sesame oil

Grilled buffalo burger on baked or grilled portabella mushroom

Mixed roasted vegetables: roast a combination of broccoli, cauliflower, and brussels sprouts, and season with olive oil and spices

Broiled chicken with peppers: roughly chop green, yellow, and red peppers, onions, and mushrooms; toss lightly with extra-virgin olive oil and chopped garlic, add chopped chicken, and broil in the oven until brown

Steamed veggies and rice (cauliflower, broccoli, carrots): drizzle with oil and lemon after steamed; serve over 1/2 cup wild or brown rice

Baked fish topped with tomato pesto

Roasted green beans with olive oil and spices

Grilled turkey breast with sage

Baked fish with lemon

Steamed green and yellow beans, topped with oil and spices

Steamed kale

Grilled chicken with garlic pesto: mix 2 cloves minced garlic and 1/8 cup extra-virgin olive oil with some finely chopped fresh basil or 1/2 teaspoon of dried basil; spread garlic-basil mixture on chicken breasts and allow to marinate, then grill

Grilled chicken, beef, or fish

Steamed broccoli with olive oil

Large mixed green salad with veggies of your choice, 3–4 ounces grilled chicken or fish, topped with oil, herbs, and spices of your choice

Two of my favorite meals to support detoxification are veggie soup and bone broth. Here are my easy-peasy recipes so you can prepare and enjoy these healthy meals.

VEGGIE SOUP RECIPE

In a large pot, sauté chopped carrots, celery, and onion in coconut oil until tender. Add cabbage, zucchini, parsnips, fennel, and any other nonstarchy vegetables. Fill pot with water. Add your favorite spices such as salt, pepper, turmeric, garlic, basil, or oregano. Bring to a boil, cover, and simmer for several hours, adding water as needed. For an even easier version, you can do this in a slow cooker.

Eat as much of this soup as you want. Try for at least 1 cup per day. This veggie soup is alkaline, and the turmeric and black pepper aid in the detoxification process. Soup is filling and satisfying.

BONE BROTH RECIPE

Place the bones from a cooked whole chicken in a large pot or slow cooker. Add water to cover. Add 1 tablespoon of vinegar and cook for 8–12 hours on a low simmer. Add more water as needed. When done, strain bones from liquid using a large colander. Place broth back into a saucepan or stockpot and add seasonings as desired such as turmeric, black pepper, chives, onion, or garlic. Or after straining, spoon into quart jars to refrigerate or freeze for later. (Be sure to leave room for expansion of liquids when freezing). Add seasonings when ready to heat and cook.

Optional: add veggies like carrots, celery, and onion to chicken bones when cooking for an extra nutrient boost.

Drink this broth as needed. It is full of electrolytes and is delicious to sip on as you would a cup of coffee.

R

CHAPTER 6

Rock Bottom Thyroid Reset: Phase Three

"I had hit 'rock bottom' on antidepressants, was overweight, and just plain felt crappy. I tried other diets prior and lost weight but could never maintain. That's when I started reaching for a functional medicine doctor or nutritionist. I contacted Tiffany about her programs. Well, I have now completed the eight-week program. When I struggled during the Prep Phase, Tiffany helped me tweak my diet, and I made it through. By the end of week four, I couldn't believe how well I was feeling, and I hadn't had coffee for two weeks!"

— Carla D., Austin, Texas

The Rebuild Phase: Week Five and Beyond

You did it! You've eaten wholesome, balanced meals for four weeks now. You've ditched gluten and dairy. And you've equipped yourself with the knowledge of how food affects you. From Week Five onward, paying attention to your symptoms will be critical to managing your health long-term.

The key is to listen to your body and feed it well. I've helped you get your health back on track, but soon you'll be on your own. That doesn't mean you can't come back to the basics anytime you feel overwhelmed. Now that you understand how to eat gluten- and dairy-free, you can repeat the Detox Phase without the Preparation Phase whenever healthy habits get put on hold (e.g., vacations, new career, stressful life events, etc.). You can detox as often as every three months.

By Week Five, you may be experiencing more energy, better focus, higher concentration, fewer (or zero) aches and pains, weight loss, and better rest. That said, improvement is different for everyone. If you still have pesky symptoms hanging around, more specific nutrient support may be necessary for you. We're going to take care of these needs in this chapter.

The Rebuild Phase is also the time to experiment with foods you took away during phases one and two (if you choose to). As you add these foods back into your diet one at a time, you'll note any symptoms that arise.

Now, it's possible that this jump-start into clean eating has you losing weight and feeling amazing—and you don't want to risk self-sabotage. If you want to stay away from gluten and dairy, I support you 100 percent. If you *do* plan on adding any foods back into your diet, reintroduce them one at a time according to the outline I give you in this chapter. We'll do this over the coming weeks, as some foods don't cause issues for several days after you've eaten them. Think one new food per week. This gives you plenty of time to notice if you have a bad reaction so you can identify which food is the problem. And, if you don't feel the need or want to add some of these foods back, you can do that too. This is your plan.

First, a quick reminder about beverages. I encourage you to keep your coffee intake to a minimum—one or two cups a day, depending on how caffeine affects you. Continue to avoid diet sodas and other artificially sweetened beverages and drink mixes. Stick to plain water, water with flavored stevia or monk fruit, naturally flavored unsweetened carbonated water, and caffeine-free tea.

Ready for the next phase?

Week Five: Fruit

If you stopped eating fruit, start with berries and eat one serving (about half a cup) each day for the first three days. Then increase to two servings (about one cup total) per day for the rest of the week. If you were just limiting fruits instead of cutting them out completely, you can do one cup of berries per day for the whole week.

Grab a notebook, your calendar, or a blank document on your phone or laptop and write down any changes in your symptoms or mood. Some people are *so* sensitive that fruits trigger cravings, and they get sucked back into their old habits. So we need to add fruit back slowly.

If you do experience any symptoms you're not thrilled with, stop eating fruit for the rest of the week. Going through this slow, important process will help you understand what your body needs to feel better for years to come.

Week Six: Nuts

Add nuts back in Week Six. Limit yourself to two servings a day, and pay attention to portion sizes. Nuts are notorious for triggering excessive eating. If you limited these rather than cut them out, now is the time to give yourself two servings. If you feel good by the end of the week, great! Nuts can stay in your diet long-term.

Week Seven: Beans

If concern about carbs made you skip beans for the past four weeks, Week Seven is your chance to add them back to your diet as well. Limit your serving size to half a cup every other day. Again, take note of any symptoms, and stop eating beans if you experience discomfort.

Week Eight: Dairy and Gluten

You may or may not have noticed changes when you cut out dairy. To find out if you're one of the few thyroid patients who tolerates it, this is the time to test it if you so desire. If not, that's fine, too. Just skip ahead to my instructions for reintroducing gluten.

If you do so desire and you're not feeling symptoms associated with dairy sensitivities, add one serving of dairy a day to your diet for two to three days. If you don't notice any changes, you may continue to eat dairy . . . *sparingly.* If you catch yourself clearing your throat, get stuffed up sinuses, have an upset stomach, feel bloated, or gain a few pounds, take these as signs that dairy is just not good for you.

Most Rock Bottom Wellness clients get excited about eating dairy again, especially during summer ice cream season. Some even feel tempted to play around with my phase three recommendations rather than try oat milk, coconut creamer, almond ice cream, or cashew "cheese." They reorder the food groups because of convenience or cravings. *I'm going to skip fruit and start with dairy. That way, I can join my son for ice cream after his baseball game this weekend.* This often backfires in some pretty nasty symptoms. You may be addicted to a certain food, so a mere four weeks isn't enough time to heal your underlying draw to it. That's why I recommend following this transition plan to add foods back into your diet.

When some of my clients go into Week Eight, they realize dairy was the culprit of their symptoms all along. They feel heartbroken. Please don't feel discouraged if that's you. You may learn you *can* tolerate dairy in your diet periodically—down the road. Just not right now. You won't know that if you jump from Week Four to Week Eight because you want a milkshake. If you're in a hurry to add a food back in, you may worsen your thyroid symptoms.

Now let's say, a few months from now, you're at someone's house for a cookout. They offer no dairy-free cheese or toppings. You didn't pack nondairy cheese, so you decide to eat a cheeseburger to be polite. This happens *all the time*. My hard-core clients would say, "Always be prepared. Bring your own food!" That's not realistic for most people. After several weeks of healing, you'll most likely be able to eat dairy once in a while with only a minor reaction.

Most likely. Some people find that taking dairy out of their diet makes all the difference in the world, and they have no desire to risk a backslide.

"I know how dairy affects me," one client told me when we discussed his upcoming vacation.

"Well, now that you've healed your body, one serving of dairy might not be detrimental."

"Maybe," he said. "But I think I'm at a point where . . ." He paused. "Nope. No way I'm gonna chance it. I remember what dairy did to me. It's not worth risking it. I'll find a grocery store and buy some almond ice cream if I want it bad enough!"

If this client is like most people, at some point he *will* risk it. It's okay to think, *You know what? It* is *worth it. I'm going to eat this, but I know what my consequences are going to be.* And you reach for the cheese or order the ice cream, and you know what you're in for. You've made that choice, but you know what to do afterward—eat how you want to feel. You haven't failed. You can always restart the detox. Don't let this book rule you to the point where you feel depressed. I'd rather have you risk a piece of cheesecake than be miserable! So think of phase three as you working my recommendations into your life.

Next up is gluten. If you want, add one or two servings to your diet for two to three days. Note any symptoms you experience. If you experience digestive problems or sinus congestion, that could mean gluten is a problem for you.

When I work with clients one-on-one during Week Eight and adding gluten back to their diet doesn't go well, they can feel pretty defeated because they feel like they need to start over. I help them navigate these feelings so they don't undo all the good they've done. Just because you have one or two bad days of testing food doesn't mean you've failed! Remember, the goal is to make the Rock Bottom Thyroid Reset work for your life. You don't want to rearrange your whole life forever. You *can* make gluten-free eating work for you, and you *can* deal with the ups and downs, holidays, special occasions, and stressful times life throws your way.

A client messaged me the morning I wrote this chapter. She texted, *I'm nervously giggling. After getting rid of gluten, I feel free. Fewer aches and pains. I feel so light and nimble. If I can have more of that . . . well, that's what I look forward to.* For this client, going gluten-free long-term supports how she wants to feel.

What I'm trying to impress upon you is that you've been at this for a few weeks. Your body may need more healing—a longer break from gluten—before you can tolerate toast again. This is why it's important not to be in too much of a hurry to add bread or other gluten back into your diet. I've had a couple of clients who struggle with emotional eating, who add everything back in one fell swoop within a couple of days. It never goes well. Often they get sick. Really sick. I understand—it's difficult to get perspective. Sometimes you have to take a couple of steps back to realize how far you've come. If that means you need to have grilled cheese for breakfast for a week, have grilled cheese for breakfast for a week. I won't be offended. Just know what you may be getting yourself into. Often people *know* when they will not be able to add this or that back to their diets. But the benefits of giving up a certain food category for good—not having symptoms—far outweigh any cravings. It's just not worth it anymore.

Beyond Rock Bottom: Thyroid Supplements

I wish swapping this food in and that food out was all your thyroid needed to get back to 100 percent. For some people, it is! But sometimes, that's not the case. No wonder prescription medicine is the most common way to treat thyroid disorders. It's cheap (or free, depending on your insurance), and it delivers fast results. It can also deliver some pretty fast side effects. But if you try to treat your thyroid with food alone, you'll miss out on an essential way to treat any thyroid condition—supplementation. In phase three, I help all my clients fill any and all nutritional gaps in their diet with specific supplements so we can continue to improve their thyroid—and their overall health.

Many doctors and health care professionals will argue against supplements. Whether supplements work or not is controversial, as I'm sure you know. In an ideal world, we'd get all of our nutrients from the foods we eat, right? But for people who've been following the Standard American Diet (SAD) for many years or who suffer from acute or chronic illness, food sometimes (most of the time, actually) isn't enough.

The SAD is full of processed grains and packaged products that try (but fail) to manage caloric intake, increase intake of grains and fiber, and reduce fat intake. By following these recommendations, we overeat and experience poor health. We eat poor-quality fats and foods with additives, preservatives, and synthetic colors. We're also intrigued by easy food we can make at home from a box. These are packaged to conform to typical dietary recommendations, which makes them seem like a healthy choice. In reality, they're far from it.

If that wasn't enough, modern American farming practices deplete our soil of nutrients. The produce we buy in grocery stores contains far fewer nutrients than it did a hundred or even fifty years ago. Most fruits and vegetables travel a long distance to get where we buy them. The quality and freshness decline over that time. Some of our fruits are sweeter than ever, and unnaturally so. Remember the grapple? The FDA and USDA approved a food manufacturer's idea to soak Fuji apples in concord grape "flavor"—a chemical called methyl anthranilate. It's a sweet, appealing flavor for some, but it's definitely not healthier. There are other examples of additives in our produce, which also contain fewer nutrients than they used to. Double whammy!

Conventional animal farming methods leave our meat much lower in key nutrients like zinc, omega-3s, and antioxidants. Grain-fed meat and farm-raised seafood carry more toxins than grass-fed and wild-caught alternatives. These toxins reduce your body's ability to use their nutrients. Even if you're eating as clean as you can, you can still lack essential nutrients. That's where the right supplements can save the day.

Another reason to take supplements is exercise. Yes, exercise. I was surprised when I first heard this, too. If you exercise, good for you. Keep it up. Just know that regular exercise increases your need for nutrients. That doesn't always mean you should eat more calories. When you work out, you use up nutrients like magnesium and calcium. What better way to get those back than to supplement? And forget exercise for a moment. If you have a chronic illness (or a thyroid health crisis), your nutrient demands increase regardless of how long you're on the treadmill. That's when supplementation is essential to save your health.

Now you know why supplements aren't optional. But where do you start? You can find a lot of contradictory information out there about supplements. Maybe you've heard alternative health claims on social media, TV, or from well-meaning friends about a certain pill that can cure all that ails you. For example, TV doctors made raspberry ketones, green tea, vitamin D, CoQ_{10}, and fish oil best selling supplements overnight. Do you need these or not? Every one-on-one client learns which supplements they need to support their thyroid. I'm going to offer that same service to you now.

Essential Thyroid Supplements

The right supplements are hard to find. It's important to know which ones your body needs to fill any nutrient gaps and improve at a cellular level, but even more important is taking the supplements in the first place! I'm going to make that super easy for you. All you have to do is go to www.rockbottomwellness.com/supplements, where I show you which professional-grade, tried-and-true supplements to buy so you get the highest-quality manufactured products with the most efficacy at the best price.

Probiotics

Probiotics are the good bacteria that occur naturally in your digestive system. We're born with a plethora of microbes in our GI tract. Probiotics support immune function, reduce inflammation, promote healthy digestion, produce vitamins B_{12} and K_2, and crowd out "bad" bacteria.

People with thyroid dysfunction tend to have poor gut health. Probiotic supplements help heal your gut faster than diet alone. Without them, reducing symptoms and feeling better can take much longer.

With our overzealous goal of killing any "germ" in sight with antibacterial everything, we're killing even the good bacteria in our bodies. With the advent of these antibacterial products (and antibiotic overuse), health conditions such as irritable bowel syndrome (IBS), inflammatory bowel syndrome (IBD), Crohn's disease, and ulcerative colitis (UC) are on the rise. Bottom line, our guts are hurting—and not just from symptoms of GI upset, diarrhea, and constipation. We're lacking a full spectrum of healthy bacteria in our GI tract.

When we ate whole foods from good soil and fermented foods before modern farming, we kept that healthy bacteria in our guts. Today, because of depleted soil, overused sanitation methods, overprescribed antibiotics, high sugar intake, inflammatory foods, emotional stress, alcohol, tobacco, poor sleep, and lack of exercise, our good gut bacteria is lacking. This causes dysbiosis—a condition in which the balance of the good gut bacteria (85 percent) and bad gut bacteria (less than 15 percent) gets out of whack. When this happens, it opens the door for the takeover of other types of harmful microbes like yeast (candida).

To get (and keep) more probiotics in your gut, skip the yogurt (dairy!) and instead drink kombucha, eat more fermented vegetables (like raw sauerkraut and kimchi), and drink apple cider vinegar (you can dilute up to three tablespoons a day in water or add it to your salad). Consume lots of fiber to feed your good, living bacteria—chia and flax are great sources of fiber, as are vegetables and fruits such as berries, avocados, pears, and apples. Take a good prebiotic with your meals as well!

I also recommend you take a quality probiotic supplement with a variety of strains (different probiotic strains impact your health in different ways). The label will list the different strains in a measurement called CFUs. Choose one from a company that accounts for conditions to keep probiotics alive (rather than storing them in an un-air-conditioned warehouse all summer).

Fish Oil

Most health care professionals have recommended fish oil for years, and now it's a huge market trend. I wouldn't be surprised if you could buy it at a gas station these days (but don't do that, please).

If you're not eating fatty fish like salmon, tuna, or mackerel a couple of times a week, you may need to supplement with fish oil. Fish oil is a source of the essential fatty acid omega-3, in particular EPA/DHA. Omega-3s reduce symptoms of inflammation. Anyone with autoimmune diseases will benefit from additional omega-3s.

Although the healthy omega-3s we're looking for are found in fish, so are heavy metals, pesticides, and other contaminants. That's why you need to know where your fish or fish oil supplement is sourced from as well as how the manufacturing and testing quality practices are done. Many fish oils you can buy over the counter are synthetic but can still be labeled as "natural triglyceride" (the best form) even if it only contains a small amount. Have you ever taken a fish oil supplement and burped the aftertaste of fish afterward? If so, then you know you have a synthetic supplement. These lesser quality fish oils can cause inflammation—the opposite of what you want! Don't worry, I'll tell you in a moment how to find a good quality fish oil.

Calcium

Calcium is the most abundant mineral found in the body. Almost 99 percent of your body's calcium is stored in your bones and teeth. This stored calcium is released into the bloodstream when it's needed for not just bone health but also for nerve transmission, blood clotting, hormonal secretion, and muscle contraction.

"How do I get calcium if I don't drink milk?" I get asked this *all* the time. High calcium foods include bok choy, kale, broccoli, okra, sardines, almonds, and spinach. It's not uncommon to have insufficient calcium due to that pesky Standard American Diet. But even when you follow a restricted diet due to food intolerance or health conditions, you can be at greater risk for calcium deficiency.

As a supplement, the form of calcium you take matters. I suggest forms of the actual vitamins and minerals that are better for absorption and assimilation by the body. Vitamin D also improves calcium absorption, so choose a calcium supplement that has vitamin D with it (or take a separate vitamin D supplement at the same time—I'll go over this soon). I suggest 1,000 mg/day, and for those older than fifty, 1,200 mg/day is better. Take your calcium at a different time of day than your thyroid medicine—otherwise, the combination may interfere with your body's ability to absorb the calcium.

Even if you take a calcium supplement with vitamin D, you also need adequate levels of magnesium to absorb calcium. (Magnesium is another bone-supportive mineral, which I'll go over next.) In nature, calcium is never found without magnesium.

Some prescription thyroid treatments cause bone density loss. If you're taking thyroid medication, eat high-calcium foods or take a supplement. Humans absorb 30 percent of the calcium found in foods, and that number decreases with age.

Magnesium

Magnesium is a critical mineral found in many functions of the body. It's not uncommon to have magnesium deficiencies due to our SAD. Alcohol and caffeine consumption along with stress all deplete your body's magnesium. Deficiencies in magnesium are associated with goiters (as seen in Graves' disease) and other complications.

Magnesium is known to support the thyroid gland in two ways. First, it helps produce more T4 (the inactive thyroid hormone). Second, it helps the conversion of T4 to T3 (the active thyroid hormone). Magnesium's job in the body also involves developing bones and teeth; metabolizing carbohydrates, fats, proteins, and blood glucose; forming cells and tissues; maintaining muscle function; producing healthy bowel movements; and maintaining your immune system and neurological health.

Food sources of magnesium include green veggies, beans, peas, nuts, seeds, and whole unprocessed grains. If you take a magnesium supplement, be sure to get the chelated form for better absorption and assimilation. You can also buy a supplement that has calcium, magnesium, and vitamin D together—just make sure both the calcium and magnesium are chelated forms.

Selenium

Selenium is a somewhat obscure mineral you don't hear much about unless you're struggling with thyroid disease. Selenium supports your immune system, reduces inflammation, and converts thyroid hormones. Selenium deficiency can cause classic hypothyroid symptoms such as fatigue, depression, and weight gain as well as sore muscles and a weakened immune system.

Food sources of selenium include Brazil nuts, brewer's yeast, liver, cold-water fish, shellfish, garlic, whole grains, and sunflower seeds. If you take a supplement, I recommend 200 mcg of selenium a day in the form of selenomethionine or selenium glycinate.

Zinc

Zinc supports your immune system, heals wounds, fosters normal fetal growth and development during pregnancy, and benefits your taste, smell, and vision. But if you take too much zinc, your copper levels can become deficient. That's why you'll often find zinc as an ingredient in other supplements in the right proportion. Over time, zinc deficiency shows up as fatigue, dermatitis, acne, loss of taste, poor wound healing, anorexia, hair loss, fingernail white spots, and night blindness. Zinc also plays a role in insulin insensitivity, which is at the core of the Rock Bottom Thyroid Reset.

To get more zinc in your diet, eat oysters, red meat, poultry, beans, and nuts. If you don't love these foods, supplementation is an option. I recommend a zinc chelate or citrate for optimal absorption, ideally combined with copper. Always take your zinc supplement with food, as it can cause nausea on an empty stomach.

Vitamin D

Most of us are deficient in vitamin D. If your doctor orders a serum test of your vitamin D, just know that these levels can fluctuate daily and don't tell you what's going on at the cellular level. That said, vitamin D is *so* important! It plays a role in maintaining a healthy immune system and proper hormone levels, promoting neuromuscular function and bone health, and keeping inflammation down. Deficiencies are linked to poor sleep and sleep apnea. It does so much and we struggle to get it, especially if you're living in a temperate climate farther from the equator. That's because the main way our bodies get vitamin D is from exposing bare skin (without sunscreen) to the sun.

Great vitamin D food sources include fatty fish like mackerel and salmon, egg yolks, and beef liver. If you're like me and you don't like fish *or* beef liver, you can take a supplement. I recommend (and use myself) a liquid drop vitamin D_3 supplement. It's easy to dose and absorb. Thyroid patients quite often have gut health issues, and absorbing nutrients can be even more difficult for them. This liquid drop form is very effective at increasing vitamin D levels.

Multivitamins and Multiminerals

Multivitamins and multiminerals are designed to be broad-spectrum supplements to fill in the nutrient gaps we have due to inadequate food choices, illness, intense exercise, or stress. You can get a multivitamin that also contains some minerals, or you can get a separate multimineral supplement. The goal of a multi is to increase your level of these micronutrients (vitamins, minerals, antioxidants, and often complementary herbs). Simple as that.

Multivitamins are a maintenance dose of nutrients that can cover these bases. I often recommend these, but you may still need to complement them with more of another nutrient. For my clients, I do in-depth vitamin and mineral testing; then I make recommendations specific to each person's results. Multis are an efficient way to get a vast array of nutrients in your diet. But no one supplement will correct everything.

When I recommend a multivitamin, I look at nutrient bioavailability (most effective for your body to use), nutrient form, and any "other ingredients." Make sure you take your multi at least four hours before or after any prescriptions. Taken at the wrong time, multivitamins can inhibit medicine absorption, disrupt your lab work, and worsen your thyroid symptoms.

What's Important When Buying Supplements?

Now that you know what supplements to take, where do you buy them? A health food store? Online? The corner drugstore? As you might guess, the most important factor to consider when choosing your brand of supplements is quality. Many of my clients once believed that all supplements were created equal. *So not true.* Most vitamin companies tout their brand as the best. As if supplements weren't confusing enough! Did you know that vitamins and supplements are unregulated? Because nobody holds any of these companies accountable, it can be difficult to figure out who to trust.

Of course, cost can be a big factor when you decide to purchase supplements. Quality supplements cost more than generic versions from the big box stores. But your body will utilize the higher-quality supplements better because of the greater bioavailability, so you'll need to take less of them over time. You may benefit from several supplements, but you'll only have to take them short-term. If you're using a low-quality version, you could take them forever and still not replenish the nutrients your body needs. The buy-one-get-one-free fish oil will cost you more in the long run because you'll have to take twice the dose to get half the benefits.

Before you add one more supplement on your credit card, I want to set the record straight. Supplementation is meant for a limited therapeutic time. You do not need to buy these for the rest of your life. I'm sorry if this is the first time you've seen this news, but it's true. Big box stores don't want you to know—they'd rather you buy their arsenic-laden, lead-laden protein powders for years and years.[2] Even without the poison, most protein shakes aren't good for you anyway. They often include genetically modified (GMO) soy, isolates, creatine, and other inflammatory ingredients that cause gastrointestinal issues. All for $130 a month. Just because it's more expensive at the store doesn't mean it's better. One of my most recommended proteins is a clean, three-ingredient powder with a month's worth of meals for $70.

Besides price, what makes one supplement better than another? The grade, form, purity, bioavailability, and third-party verification all contribute to the effectiveness of a product. Nutritional supplements

---

[2] Jesse Hirsch, "Arsenic, Lead Found in Popular Protein Supplements," *Consumer Reports*, March 12, 2018, www.consumerreports.org/dietary-supplements/heavy-metals-in-protein-supplements/.

are available in different grades. These grades include pharmaceutical and cosmetic (or nutritional grade). Pharmaceutical grade is the highest-quality grade of vitamins. It means the purity, dissolution, and absorption meets the highest regulatory standard verified by an outside party. This grade has undergone third-party quality and efficacy verification testing. The manufacturer produces all their own products, so they know where they come from. Quality-control measures are utilized with each individual package (versus exposing a whole batch to irradiation when a "bug" is found, then selling it even though it's less effective). Some pharmaceutical-grade supplements are available without a prescription, but they're sold by health care practitioners such as functional nutritionists like me.

Cosmetic- or nutritional-grade supplements are sold in most health food stores, online, and through direct sales companies. These supplements might not always be tested for absorption, dissolution, or purity. They don't always have the same concentrations of active ingredients listed on the label. Remember, this industry is not regulated, so what's on the label isn't always what's in the bottle. Comparison studies show that direct sales brands and drugstore brands don't hold up to the quality and efficacy of pharmaceutical- and professional-grade supplements.

Why all these standards and comparisons? Why does purity, form, and bioavailability matter? Well, for example, if you have GI issues on top of a thyroid disorder, one form of vitamin D may work better for you than another. If you're taking synthetic vitamin E versus natural vitamin E, you won't absorb it as well through the digestive tract. One form of magnesium acts as a laxative and can leave you with GI issues, whereas other forms help your heart, muscles, sleep, and nervous system. All supplements should be screened for pesticides, mercury, lead, and other toxic ingredients—but many aren't. In fact, several fish oils on the market have been found to contain mercury, which can build up and harm your brain, heart, kidneys, and lungs.

To avoid these problems, I recommend you go with pharmaceutical-grade supplements. If you can't find the supplement you want to purchase in a pharmaceutical grade, choose one that is Good Manufacturing Practice (GMP) certified, at minimum. There are other standards some supplement companies use to provide even more purity, efficacy, and quality. You can also see if they perform laboratory analysis and disintegration studies on their products. While it's possible to find high-quality supplements on your own (and with the help of this book), the easiest and most direct way is to seek out a certified nutritionist to get the best quality for your specific needs.

If you'd like to skip the tedious, time-consuming supplement research process, head over to www.rockbottomwellness.com/supplements, where I show you the most up-to-date list of supplement products and where to order them at the best price.

Supplements and Your Thyroid: A Cautionary Tale

When you're taking thyroid medicine (or any medication), you need to have someone guiding you who understands the interaction between different nutrients and medication. As mentioned, some minerals can block the absorption of thyroid medications.

After my cancer treatment, I worked with a professional who knew my prescriptions, my cancer, and my struggles. She recommended my supplements, and I took them religiously. The next time I had my thyroid numbers checked, they were all awful. My tumor markers and my TSH had gone up, meaning I felt dead tired.

My medicine wasn't working because I was taking several (healthy, good quality) minerals that blocked the absorption of thyroid medicine. So please, don't learn this lesson for yourself. If you have a thyroid condition, you can't just go off what someone says on a radio or TV commercial. You have to know the when, the how, and the why. For me, this was a medication/supplement timing issue that both of us failed to consider. I will not make that mistake again.

And now you won't either.

R

CHAPTER 7

Why Doesn't My Family Care? And Other Thyroid Questions Google Can't Answer

"You have done so much for my mental and physical health. The kids say I am much happier and not as stressed. Everyone is asking what I've changed because I am so much more happy, showing the weight loss, and just glowing. I hand them your business card and say, 'Tiffany truly changed my life—give her a call!'"

— Harriet C., St. Paul, Minnesota

You've learned about nutrition. You've reset your thyroid. You've learned the basics about vitamins and supplements. Now what? Is everything in your life magically "fixed"? If only. Even if we eat the best foods, take the right supplements, and exercise often, life throws curveballs when you least expect them. Depression. Stress. Autoimmune disease. Or worse.

Our bodies are complicated. What affects one organ affects everything else. If all I talked about was thyroid, thyroid, thyroid, I wouldn't be telling you everything you need to know. How nutrition impacts your health isn't the *only* thing you want to learn anyway, right? My clients worry about everything from their cholesterol to intermittent fasting to family dinners with gluten in every dish.

That's why I'm dedicating an entire chapter to answering the most common health questions I hear from clients. The ones that you can't just google. Well, you try to look them up, but you won't find an answer you can trust. Visit one web page, read something, visit another page, read the exact opposite. Not very helpful, is it? That's what this chapter will be—helpful.

If a topic doesn't apply to you right now, feel free to skip ahead to the next one, making a mental note to come back to that page when it does. Everybody sleeps, of course, but some people don't struggle to find a supportive exercise routine. That's okay. Take what works, skip what doesn't. Let's dive in.

"How do I stop being so stressed all the time?"

Stress can be good or bad. *Good stress? How is that a thing?* Glad you asked. For many people, good stress comes around the holidays, a time of happiness, family, and memories. Yet the planning, shopping, baking, traveling, and sometimes family put undue stress on our body. This "good" stress weakens our immune system, makes us munch on unhealthy foods, and sets us up to get sick.

Your body doesn't care what caused the stress. It responds the same way—fight or flight. Life never gives us a break from stress, so our adrenal glands step up to help manage it. Our adrenals soak up any B vitamins and vitamin C in our body like crazy. There aren't many of those nutrients left for other bodily functions that require them.

So, how do you support your body through stress besides taking your vitamins? How do you make *you* a priority? Finding balance in this day and age is no easy task. We have so many obligations on our schedules. Remembering what's important (our health) needs to be a concerted effort. Because when you balance your emotions, you balance your thyroid. It's that simple. When your thyroid hormones are imbalanced, stress settles into the body. Your thyroid stresses out, then you feel stressed out, making your thyroid more stressed. On and on the vicious cycle goes. Let this stress persist, and over time, you'll develop chronic illness. Any health complications are our bodies telling us we need to rest. But most of us just keep going . . . like the Energizer bunny. It's hard to stop and rest until sickness or fatigue leave us no choice. I'm not going to let you get to that point. You're going to find balance *now.*

Practical De-Stress Tips for Busy People

"Just relax!"

Yeah, right. Easier said than done. Lucky for you, you have a head start on stress relief—the Rock Bottom Thyroid Reset. You're eating to support your body. Now let's add some self-care. Do just *one* thing for yourself each day and you'll help yourself through stressful times. If you're at a loss for what self-care could look like for you, borrow these tips. Here are my favorite strategies you can use today to keep yourself feeling balanced.

Meditate. A Massachusetts General Hospital study found that regular meditation helped people feel calmer and less stressed.[3] Now, I get that sitting cross-legged with your eyes closed doesn't

---

[3] Brigid Schulte, "Harvard Neuroscientist: Meditation Not Only Reduces Stress, Here's How It Changes Your Brain," *Washington Post,* May 26, 2015, https://www.washingtonpost.com/news/inspired-life/wp/2015/05/26/harvard-neuroscientist-meditation-not-only-reduces-stress-it-literally-changes-your-brain/.

appeal to everyone. Nor is it practical. You can't chant your mantra out loud during a stressful business meeting! That's why you should find fifteen to thirty minutes every day to just *be*. Let yourself regroup and re-center. For you, meditation might look like a power nap, prayer, a few yoga poses, calming music, or a walk outside on your break. Whatever you do, make sure the activity goes in your calendar. No excuses now!

Eat whole foods and lots of them. That's what this book is for! Besides the Rock Bottom Thyroid Reset meal ideas, you can fix a big batch of soup on weekends so you can have easy, hot meals during the week. Keep quick salad ingredients in your fridge at all times. Eat citrus, strawberries, and bell peppers for a vitamin C boost. Get your B vitamins from seeds and quality animal products. If you ever feel overwhelmed or slip into SAD eating habits, refer back to this book to "reset" your sense of balance.

Exercise. Adding physical activity to your routine helps your body handle stress. I'm sure you know how regular exercise makes you feel. The chemicals your body produces give you a better outlook on life, don't they? Maintain some kind of exercise program to feel like that every day. Any form of exercise counts, whether it's your favorite group exercise class, a walk on the treadmill or outside, a stroll through the mall with your kids, running the vacuum, gardening, mowing the lawn, playing sports, biking to work, or taking a yoga class. Which brings me to my next tip . . .

Do yoga. Yoga is mental as much as physical. You wouldn't believe what even *one* class per week can do for your strength, flexibility, and peace of mind. Find a class that fits your schedule and your family—an evening class, partner yoga, or mommy-and-me yoga. Can't find the time to get away from home or the office?

Check out easy yoga routines online and follow along on your yoga mat in front of the TV.

Sleep. Easy to skip that extra hour when you wake up early, isn't it? Restful sleep is a top priority during stressful seasons of life. I mean actual restorative sleep. Get to bed and wake up at the same time every night and morning. Set a strict bedtime for yourself like the one you had when you were six. If your alarm goes off at 6:00 a.m., have a mandatory "lights out" time at 10:00 p.m. every night. No matter what. It's easier to stick to when your partner helps you enforce it. If you find falling asleep hard, try my next tip fifteen minutes before bed.

Enjoy progressive relaxation. Focus your mind on each part of your body. One part at a time. From your toes all the way up to your head. Contract your muscles, hold, then release. You're relaxing everything. Do this at bedtime and you'll fall asleep before you know it.

Remove toxins. I mean both chemical toxins like those found in processed foods, commercial health and beauty items, and cleaning supplies as well as toxic relationships. Stress from toxic products and people can keep you sick.

Treat yourself. A massage. A facial. Anything that makes your body feel good. Make it a regular scheduled date with yourself!

Use the essentials. I use essential oil blends on a daily basis. My favorite is a blend of spruce, frankincense, and blue tansy. I rub the oil on the bottom of my feet after I shower. I also add a couple of drops behind my ears (where the vagus nerve is) and at the center of my chest near my heart. Any oil with a pleasant aroma will work.

"Is my thyroid the reason I'm depressed?"

Can you relate to any of these?

● Suffering a depressed mood most of the day, every day

● Diminished interest in activities

● Significant weight loss (when not dieting) or weight gain

● Sleeping more than usual or having difficulty sleeping

● Feeling fatigued every day

● Feeling worthless or guilty

● Having difficulty concentrating or making decisions

● Thinking about death or attempting suicide

If you're contemplating self-harm or suicide and you live in the United States, know that you're not alone. Confidential help is available for free. Call the National Suicide Prevention Lifeline at 1-800-273-8255 for 24/7 confidential support. If you do not live in the USA, google "suicidal thoughts help" for instant help in your country.

The fact is, an imbalanced thyroid can be to blame for many cases of depression. The association between thyroid function and mental health, particularly with mood disorders, was recognized two hundred years ago! We've found medical reports from 1825 documenting "nervous affections" in thyroid patients.[4] In 1949, physician Richard Asher coined the term "myxedema madness" to describe the mental

---

[4] Mirella P. Hage and Sami T. Azar, "The Link between Thyroid Function and Depression," *Journal of Thyroid Research* 2012 (December 14, 2011), https://www.hindawi.com/journals/jtr/2012/590648/.

condition of people suffering with hypothyroidism.[5] In plain English, the fact is that people with thyroid issues have a higher risk of mood and anxiety disorders. A reported four in ten people with depression have a thyroid problem.[6] Because most thyroid conditions go undiagnosed, I imagine the actual number to be much higher.

What to Do About It

What can you do if you're struggling with depression *and* a thyroid condition? You're reading this book, and that's a great start. You can also advocate for yourself at every doctor's appointment. Adding thyroid medications like Synthroid (generic name: levothyroxine) to antidepressants is not accepted in mainstream medicine. However, it could be a viable treatment. It was for me. That's why you need to pay attention to your symptoms, even by writing them down in a journal. Then find a doctor who cares about how you feel—or thank goodness if yours already does.

Depression is often treated on a few reported symptoms. Rarely do doctors listen to your heart, run blood tests, monitor your pulse, or look at outward symptoms to understand what's happening on the inside. During the typical depression evaluation, you don't get asked about what you eat or what toxins you may have been exposed to. Suboptimal thyroid function is a common cause of depression, but doctors miss this if their first course of action is a prescription rather than blood tests and a treatment strategy to improve your thyroid hormone levels. Medications most often used for depression include

---

[5] Thomas W. Heinrich, MD, and Garth Grahm, MD, Hypothyroidism Presenting as Psychosis: Myxedema Madness Revisited," *Primary Care Companion to the Journal of Clinical Psychiatry* 5, no. 6 (2003): 260–266.
[6] Mirella and Page, "Link," https://www.hindawi.com/journals/jtr/2012/590648/.

SSRIs, MAOIs, SNRIs, and various antianxiety medications. These increase the levels of different neurotransmitters (brain chemicals), consequently improving symptoms. That's the hope, anyway.

As you can imagine, I help thyroid patients with depression all the time. Depression affects everyone differently, but I've seen many people make dramatic improvements once we got them eating right and supplementing smart. One such supplement is vitamin B_{12}. A study on depression found that patients who received B_{12} injections improved significantly.[7] Another common nutritional deficiency among thyroid patients with depression is fatty acids. Research indicates that depression may be linked to chronic inflammation.[8] If so, addressing a fatty acid imbalance could solve the underlying *physical* problem manifesting as a psychological one. More omega-3s, improved neuronal communication, better mood.

Some people respond to nutritional interventions alone. Others may find that particular nutrients may help improve the effect of antidepressants that were otherwise unhelpful. If you're taking medications to treat depression, your nutrient deficiencies can be *worse* than if you took no prescription at all. Replenish your body where you're deficient, and medications often work better. I've also seen people test how they feel on and off medications. (Always do this under the supervision of your doctor.)

---

[7] Ehsan Ullah Syed, Mohammad Wasay, and Safia Awan, "Vitamin B12 Supplementation in Treating Major Depressive Disorder: A Randomized Controlled Trial," *Open Neurology Journal* 7 (November 15, 2013): 44–48.

[8] Andrew H. Miller and Charles L. Raison, "The Role of Inflammation in Depression: From Evolutionary Imperative to Modern Treatment Target," *Nature Review Immunology* 16, no. 1 (January 2016): 22–34.

Either way, I have no idea why mainstream health practitioners don't see the connection between what we put in our body and what happens in our mind. Believe it or not, the head is attached to the body. Yes, most antidepressants deal with the brain's neurotransmitters, but why don't we consider nutritional deficiencies? Our body and our mind work together, so they should be treated that way.

Just as no two people have the same body or mind, no two depression diagnoses are alike. When you weed out the varying symptoms of depression, they lump roughly into four categories. Depending on which category of depression you have, there are other specific strategies that can help you overcome what you're going through so you can start feeling like yourself again.

The Four Categories of Depression (and Their Action Plans)

Read the bullet statements, add up the total number that apply to you, and move on to the Action Plan for your "brand" of depression. Each Action Plan explains the specific reasons behind your symptoms and what you can do about them.

Depression Type #1: In the Dark

Which points resonate with you? If several apply, check out the information on what may be causing these feelings.

● Would people describe you as an overall negative person?

● Do you feel worried or anxious much of the time?

● Do you have low self-esteem, feel guilty, or are often self-critical?

● Is it hard to turn your mind off at night from negative thoughts?

● Are you a perfectionist? Inflexible? A control freak?

● Are you just plain *sad?*

● Do you avoid hot weather?

● Do you use sweets, caffeine, or alcohol in the evenings to calm down?

● Do you have unexplained muscle or joint pain?

● Have you benefited from antidepressants that target serotonin?

● Do you tend to get more energy at night or stay up late?

● Does exercise give you some relief from this dark feeling?

● Do you suffer from tears and anger related to your period?

What to Do If You're in the Dark

All of these symptoms are different versions of feeling like you're under a dark cloud. On top of depression, you may also experience panic, insomnia, irritability, PMS, and muscle pain. You likely have a serotonin deficiency.

Serotonin is a neurotransmitter that helps you maintain a positive mood, good sleep habits, and satiety. Serotonin needs to fire at all times if you're going to feel well and whole. Don't have enough serotonin, and those happy feelings tank.

Serotonin is produced in our body by an amino acid called tryptophan. You've probably heard tryptophan associated with the sleepy effect from Thanksgiving turkey dinner. You'll find it in other foods like beef and cheese as well—high quality, of course. Tryptophan converts into another amino acid, 5-HTP, which then converts into serotonin.

Sometimes medications designed to boost serotonin can make things somewhat better, but the results tend to be limited. Serotonin boosters may take the edge off but not fix the underlying issue. Some clients tell me they're told to stay on their medication even though their meds don't make them feel better.

Whether you're on medication or not, you can be proactive about boosting your serotonin. Low calories and skipped meals deplete your serotonin stores. To get those serotonin levels up, protein is the name of the game. Get about four ounces of quality animal protein at every meal and about half that at each snack. If you're a vegetarian or vegan, include foods such as nutritional yeast, nuts, seeds, pumpkin, and bananas in your diet.

You also need healthy dietary fats like olive oil, avocado oil, coconut oil, butter, and ghee. Healthy fats increase the bioavailability of tryptophan in the brain. That's why low-fat diets cause anger and a negative attitude. It's that serotonin deficiency! Meanwhile, avoid low-quality fats like vegetable oils, margarine, and other processed oils.

While you're eating that grass-fed, gluten-free burger cooked in avocado oil, add whole, fresh foods on the side. A serotonin-deficient body needs vitamins and minerals such as calcium, magnesium, B vitamins, vitamin C, and vitamin D. Stress is a common serotonin zapper, using up the B vitamins and vitamin C that support the adrenals. I find people with depression are often deficient in vitamin B_6, specifically. Vitamin B_6 is basically the raw material for making serotonin.

To help relieve that stress, get moving! You don't have to kill yourself at the gym to help mitigate symptoms of depression. When you exercise, your muscles demand more amino acids to help repair tissue. That's when tryptophan gets sent right to the brain to help make serotonin. Increased oxygen also increases your serotonin.

Getting out to exercise for even thirty minutes can boost your mood.

In the Dark Action Plan

● Eat 4 ounces of protein at each meal.

● Eat healthy fats.

● Manage your stress. Eat a lot of B vitamin and vitamin C foods.

● Eat whole, fresh food.

● Exercise 30 minutes per day.

Depression Type #2: Who Cares?

Which points resonate with you? If several apply, check out the information on what may be causing these feelings.

● Do you often feel bored, apathetic, or flat?

● Do you have low mental or physical energy?

● Do you have low motivation?

● Do you sleep a lot more than what would be considered "normal"?

● Do you put on weight easily?

● Do you consume a lot of caffeine, chocolate, or other stimulants to stay awake or motivated?

What to Do If You Don't Care

You don't care enough to focus. You don't care enough to enjoy anything that used to make you happy. And you don't care enough about that to get angry. You just don't care.

If this description fits your depression, you may have a catecholamine deficiency. The three catecholamines are dopamine, norepinephrine, and adrenaline. Dopamine is king—it creates the other two. Together, these chemicals make you feel energized and excited emotionally, physically, and mentally. Catecholamines also affect your adrenal gland function. Again, everything in our body is connected.

Everyone has had an adrenaline rush or felt that fight-or-flight response. Anything, really, can trigger a catecholamine response. Anticipation of a meal, a vacation, a presentation you're about to give, or being stuck in traffic. Whatever you feel in each situation is the result of catecholamine release.

If your catecholamines are low, you feel stuck. Your reaction time slows. You're distracted. And you don't care. Stimulants like caffeine, chocolate, tobacco, or artificial sweeteners have a temporary effect. You reach for more and more, but you don't feel "up."

Have you felt prolonged stress or suffered through a terrible illness? These are other reasons why you feel bogged down, fatigued, apathetic, and distracted. After a while, your brain can't keep up with the body's demand for catecholamine, and your adrenal glands slow down. You burn out and pretty much don't care about a thing.

Similar to "in the dark" depression, you need animal protein and omega-3s. Amino acids produce both serotonin and catecholamines. In this case, the amino acid is tyrosine. Protein malnutrition is a major cause of feeling apathetic long-term. This won't feel intuitive. People with type #2 depression feel drawn to high-carb, high-sugar, and high-starch food. These deplete your catecholamines because insulin is released, which pulls amino acids into your muscles rather than your brain. Not good. Again, animal protein. Animal protein contains more tyrosine than vegetable protein (800 mg in three eggs versus 150 mg in twenty-five almonds). Low-quality soy protein inhibits tyrosine conversion into catecholamines.

If you're already depleted in catecholamines, you may not have the energy to exercise. It's a catch-22. If you feel so low that exercise makes you feel worse, or you can't even get to that point, don't push yourself. Work on nutrition first; then add light exercise such as walking, yoga, or Pilates. Even reading a book under a tree is helpful. Relaxing activities like these help your body produce the catecholamines your brain needs.

Who Cares Action Plan

- Eat 4–5 ounces of quality animal protein at each meal and half that at snacks to increase your tyrosine.

- Consider tyrosine supplementation. (Talk with a health care practitioner to ensure safety when adding this supplement. Tyrosine can be tricky when taken with prescription meds.)

- Eat regularly. Don't skip meals or restrict calories to less than 1,200 per day.

- Increase your B vitamins, iron, zinc, and selenium intake.

- Reduce or eliminate soy-based foods.

- Monitor and manage stress.

Depression Type #3: Hypersensitivity

Which points resonate with you? If several apply, check out the information on what may be causing these feelings.

- Do people see you as sensitive? Does emotional pain cause issues in every aspect of your life?

- Do you cry over just about anything?

● Do you avoid dealing with difficult issues?

● Have you been through a great deal of emotional or physical pain?

● Do you look for pleasure and comfort from sweets, starches, alcohol, or drugs?

● Is it hard to get over loss?

What to Do If You're Hypersensitive

Do you know people who take pleasure in everything life offers? Do you also know people who are always sad for no apparent reason? Happy people rebound from life's disappointments, but the people who feel low seem to carry that burden forever. It's all because of endorphins. Or lack of them. People who thrive have a great supply of these wonderful mood-boosting chemicals. If life always sucks, your endorphins are low. Endorphins keep you from feeling too much pain and calm you down by decreasing your cortisol.

Are you the hypersensitive type? If so, you might compensate for low endorphins by building an emotional wall. You may also look for comfort in sweet and fatty foods as well as in alcohol, drugs, or sex. Yes, all these can increase your endorphins. So can exercise and meditation. It's human nature to go with the path of least resistance . . . meaning eat bad foods, drink alcohol, and abuse drugs.

How did you get here? Well, you could have been born this way. Maybe family and friends called you a crybaby long after your infant years. Do you have a hard time coming out of disappointment? Do you have a family history of comfort food and substance abuse? If so, the cause could be your genes.

Or maybe not. Are you burdened by chronic stress? Prolonged and relentless problems in life? Every time you're sick, injured, under pressure, or grieving, you deplete your endorphin supply. Women have lower endorphin levels as they move through the hormone cycles of life.

My recommendations for what to do about hypersensitivity are pretty much the same as the first two depression types. Animal protein, healthy fats, whole foods, and proper supplementation send your endorphin levels back up where they should be.

Hypersensitivity Action Plan

● Eat 4–5 ounces of protein at each meal to boost amino acids.

● Increase fresh vegetable intake.

● Eat healthy fats.

● Take a quality multivitamin and multimineral.

● Consider supplementation of D and L forms of the amino acid phenylalanine. (Talk with a health care practitioner to ensure safety when adding this supplement. Phenylalanine can be tricky or exacerbate conditions if you're on medication for a thyroid condition, depression, or other issues.)

Depression Type #4: Tired and Wired

Which points resonate with you? If several apply, check out the information on what may be causing these feelings.

● Do you feel pressured and overwhelmed all the time?

● Do you have trouble relaxing?

● Are you easily upset or frustrated?

● Are you sensitive to things like bright light, noise, or fumes?

● Do you feel worse if you skip meals?

● Do you use food, alcohol, or drugs to relax?

What to Do If You're Tired and Wired

If you feel overwhelmed, overburdened, or edgy, you probably fall into this category. When you can't cope with stress—even "normal" stress—you have adrenal burnout. All stress triggers the same response. First, adrenaline alerts you to the "danger." Second, cortisol subdues the adrenaline rush and gives you strength and stamina to get through the situation. Bombard yourself with stress, and you deplete your adrenaline to the point where you feel depressed, tired, and anxious all the time.

This is that classic "being constantly chased by the saber-toothed tiger" feeling so many of us have in this modern-day society. Our body isn't designed to deal with relentless stress. Like anything else we don't take care of, the body breaks down. As a result, you're sensitive to smells and noises. You get sick easily. You don't feel rested upon waking. You *need* caffeine. You get brain fog. You can't get over that heartburn. You feel weak and can't breathe well. You grind your teeth. Don't expect your health to improve if you don't take care of the problem yourself. Yes, you need animal protein and healthy fats, but you also need specific brain-boosting supplements.

Tired and Wired Action Plan

● Consider supplementing with the brain's version of Valium— it's called GABA.

● Consider supplementing with the amino acid glycine. This relaxes your muscles even more than GABA.

● Consider supplementing with another type of amino acid, taurine, which soothes your nerves.

● Eat healthy fats.

● Eat 4–6 ounces of animal protein at every meal and half that for snacks.

● Eat healthy carbohydrates—that means whole foods.

"Which thyroid tests should I do?"

When you're trying to get to the bottom of your health concerns, conventional thyroid testing just gets in your way. Typical thyroid lab tests at your doctor's office like TSH and T4 often show nothing wrong *despite* ongoing, often debilitating symptoms. Why? Because these basic tests have such a wide range for "normal" results that you have to be sick before any problems show.

If your ongoing symptoms could be attributed to a thyroid disorder, seek out a practitioner who is open to a full panel of thyroid tests. I recommend several specific tests, which will assess how well your thyroid is functioning as well as give you information to combat your thyroid symptoms and your depression. As you know, these symptoms overlap.

Free T3

T3 is the main thyroid hormone that regulates metabolism and growth throughout the body. It's more potent than T4, affecting the heart, blood vessels, bones, muscles, and brain. T3 increases the body's metabolic rate, controls body temperature, regulates neurotransmitter synthesis (mood), impacts heart rate, and oversees food conversion into energy.

Free T4

Considered a precursor hormone, T4 is converted into T3 as required by the body's cells. Generally, this conversion occurs outside the thyroid in the liver and kidneys. Although T4 is more abundant in the blood than T3, it is less potent.

TSH

Also known as thyrotropin, TSH (thyroid-stimulating hormone) tells the thyroid to increase or decrease production of T4 or conversion to T3 depending on the amounts of T4 and T3 circulating in the bloodstream. TSH levels are high when thyroid function is poor or inefficient (hypothyroidism). Conversely, low TSH indicates an overactive thyroid (hyperthyroidism).

Thyroglobulin

The main function of thyroglobulin (Tg) is to store iodine, a nutrient necessary to produce the thyroid hormones T3 and T4. It is a protein found in the thyroid. Monitor your Tg levels over time. Don't take a single measurement. Why? Because Tg is a good indication of disease processes that affect thyroid function as well as a useful tumor marker, especially in patients with previous thyroid cancer. Guess who gets her Tg tested once a year?

TG Antibodies

The presence of antibodies to thyroglobulin (a precursor to T4) suggests an abnormal immune response against your own body, also called autoimmunity. Specifically, anti-Tg suggests a person's immune system is attacking healthy tissue—in this case, the protein precursor to thyroid hormone.

TPO Antibodies

Thyroid peroxidase (TPO) is an enzyme that initiates the synthesis of T4. Antibodies to TPO indicate autoimmunity, meaning the body is attacking normal proteins in the blood (in this case, TPO). People with anti-TPO have a higher chance of developing hypothyroidism than those without TPO antibodies.

Reverse T3

As the name implies, reverse T3 (rT3) opposes the biological action of T3. This hormone slows metabolism and renders T3 in the body biologically inactive. The rT3 production rate relative to T3 increases when you're stressed, you have nutrient deficiencies, you're experiencing inflammation, or your body doesn't agree with a certain medication.

"What about celiac disease, lupus, and other autoimmune problems?"

Inflammation is a normal, healthy response to an injury suffered by the body. For example, when there is a cut in your skin, white blood cells rush to the rescue and get rid of any foreign invaders to avoid causing an infection. The outward appearance is redness and swelling around the site. Beneath the surface is a flurry of activity for the body's protection.

Chronic inflammation is another story. When we bombard our bodies with stress, a poor diet, illness, and medications, your tissues inflame. It's a basic survival instinct. Because this inflammatory response isn't always specific, it can persist. The body can overreact to that which is harmless—*the body itself.* Cue autoimmune diseases. Many autoimmune diseases, including celiac disease and rheumatoid arthritis, are associated with chronic inflammation.

Keeping your thyroid hormones balanced isn't the only reason to avoid gluten. Often, thyroid patients have a compromised digestive tract. For this reason, you need to be aware of diseases like celiac. It is a destructive inflammatory disease of the upper small intestine mucosa resulting from gluten. Eat gluten a lot and villous atrophy occurs. That means the lining of your small intestine erodes away. The best treatment is to maintain a gluten-free diet to heal damage already done to the digestive tract's mucosal lining.

Common celiac disease and gluten-intolerance symptoms include irritable bowel syndrome, anemia, slight weight loss, inability to lose weight, and fatigue. Sometimes the disease is quiet until major destruction of the mucosal lining has occurred. If undetected long enough, the disease may worsen into malabsorption problems and secondary autoimmune diseases such as thyroiditis.

Another autoimmune disease is rheumatoid arthritis (RA), also an example of inflammation. Whatever your additional autoimmune concerns, the answer is always, always, always food. Whatever you put into your body affects what happens inside it. Decrease your inflammation and amazing things happen. Yes, that means weight loss. Water weight, fat, who cares? The goal is to keep that inflammation down. One thyroid patient brought her RA joint pain down to nothing within four weeks.

So, what can you do to avoid chronic inflammation? If you completed the Rock Bottom Thyroid Reset, you're already doing it. What we put in our bodies is key to avoiding inflammation. Adding more vegetables and fruits to the diet will increase antioxidant activity, thereby decreasing inflammatory activity. Eat a variety of colors to get the right amount of phytonutrients. You can also eat tuna, salmon, or other cold-water fish two to three times per week. Consider supplementation with quality fish oil.

Another way to lower inflammation is to avoid trans fats and sugars. These damaging fats occur naturally in some foods, but the synthetic version found in processed foods like margarine inflame tissues and damage blood vessel walls. Simple sugars, which cause chronic inflammation, can cause type-2 diabetes.

A nondietary way to improve inflammation is adequate exercise—just not too much. Beating yourself up at the gym sets the stage for stress and, yes, inflammation. A goal of thirty minutes of moderate activity every day helps stave off inflammation if you're feeling balanced.

"What should I do about my cholesterol? Stop eating saturated fat?"

Google cholesterol and saturated fat and you'll see everything from "lard is healthy" to "red meat will kill you." These are hot topics, all right. Confusing, too. What are the facts? Well, we know that the liver produces cholesterol in response to inflammation to repair our body. If inflammation is fire, cholesterol is the firefighter. A cholesterol test is called a lipid panel. When our lipid panel comes back with elevated cholesterol numbers, that's telling us (and the doctor) something. You've got inflammation! Instead of dealing with the problem, many doctors prescribe statins to bring down that cholesterol and tell you to stop eating saturated fat. Neither solution deals with the cause of inflammation. Address only the symptoms (elevated cholesterol levels) and that ongoing inflammation puts you at risk of chronic disease.

I'm not afraid of saturated fats, because they do not increase cholesterol. If you're getting saturated fat from clean, whole, and healthy food, there's no issue. Get your saturated fat from an avocado, good for you. But if you're eating a donut? Saturated trans fats from processed foods—even if they're organic, even if they're vegan—will cause problems.

Without cholesterol and saturated fats, our cells would not communicate throughout the body. Proteins would not be able to do their jobs. Cholesterol (and saturated fats) gives cells their shape and structure. Without these fats, the cell membranes would not perform their many functions.

About one-fourth of our cholesterol is in the brain. When we take statins or our cholesterol levels go under 160 or so, cognitive decline may set in. That's because cholesterol supports the nervous system. A substance on our neurons (nerve cells) called myelin helps with this transmission. Think of myelin as a protective coating. Myelin is made of cholesterol. Due to genetics or autoimmune disease, in extreme cases some people lose their myelin and develop conditions such as MS (multiple sclerosis) or ALD (adrenoleukodystrophy). Think of the movie *Lorenzo's Oil* from the 1990s.

Hormones are also made from cholesterol. Testosterone, estrogen, progesterone, pregnenolone, and androsterone are made from cholesterol. Without proper levels of these hormones, you can develop infertility, premenstrual conditions, PCOS, adrenal stress, and, yes, thyroid conditions.

Cholesterol improves digestion. In order to digest the nutrients in our foods, the liver produces bile, which is stored in the gallbladder. Bile is made from cholesterol. So, without cholesterol, we would have difficulty absorbing fats and the nutrients that are soluble in fats like vitamins A, D, E, and K.

Believe it or not, cholesterol supports immune health. Our immune system goes through the following simple process to protect us from getting infections:

1. We eat horrible processed foods. Over time, this damages our body and inflammation occurs (the fire).

2. The body recognizes this damage and tells the liver to produce cholesterol to repair the damage (the firefighters).

3. We do this over and over. The liver sends cholesterol to the inflammation resulting from poor food choices, injury, surgery, illness, etc. Arteries become clogged with cholesterol.

4. We get a lipid panel done at the doctor's office and surprise! We have high cholesterol.

5. We are prescribed statin medications to reduce cholesterol numbers without paying attention to what caused that cholesterol increase.

Maybe statins aren't the answer. What do those scary cholesterol numbers mean anyway? Besides total cholesterol and triglycerides, doctors look at low-density lipoprotein (LDL) and high-density lipoprotein (HDL). Mainstream medicine supposes that HDL is the "good" cholesterol and LDL is the "bad." You want a total cholesterol number less than 200, they say. Higher than that, and you are in danger of heart disease. That's when doctors put you on a statin. So you could conclude that too much HDL (the good kind) leads to a bad thing—total cholesterol over 200. That doesn't make sense, does it?

So let's look further into LDL and HDL. To simplify all this (not!), we need to know about something called small, dense LDL (*bad*, bad cholesterol); large, fluffy, buoyant cholesterol (*good*, bad LDL); and intermediate LDL (can be both good and bad). On top of all this, we have *good*, good cholesterol (HDL 1, HDL 2) and *bad*, good cholesterol (HDL 3). Most conventional doctors only look at total cholesterol levels, individual HDL and LDL, and triglycerides, which as you can see is missing some telling information.

Incomplete testing, incomplete solution. Remember those statin drugs? Statins block cholesterol production in the liver. Statins block several other pathways as well. One pathway is CoQ_{10}, an important nutrient for your immune system, heart health, and brain health. This may be why a very low cholesterol level can interfere with cognitive function. Why are we encouraged to take something that blocks a nutrient from doing its job?

That's not the only problem with statins. Some studies even show statins may accelerate calcium deposit into arteries instead of bones where it belongs.[9] When our arteries become blocked with calcium, bad things happen! I'm shocked that statins are now recommended across the board to people with chronic diseases such as diabetes, regardless of their cholesterol levels. This is because they are at greater risk of heart disease, which in my humble opinion is an inflammation problem, not a cholesterol problem. I have clients who complain about brain fog and joint pain but have *no* elevated cholesterol. It's yet one more reason to educate yourself so you can tell your doctor what you want to do, not the other way around.

Again, most doctors know little to nothing about nutrition. Ever heard of the Framingham Heart Study? This study followed fifteen thousand people over three generations. It showed that foods with

---

[9] "Plaque Paradox: Statins Increase Calcium in Atheromas Even as They Shrink Them," Cleveland Clinic, October 20, 2015, https://consultqd.clevelandclinic.org/plaque-paradox-statins-increase-calcium-in-coronary-atheromas-even-while-shrinking-them/.

cholesterol have no correlation to heart disease.[10] This begs the question: If we're told to eat a low-fat, whole-grain diet, why do we need these statins? Not to prevent heart attacks, that's for sure. Did you know that 75 percent of heart attack patients have *normal* cholesterol?[11] Probably not. Because mainstream medicine doesn't tell you. So while you're reading up on the truth, know that you can reach for that avocado guilt-free. *Bon appétit!*

"How do I get more sleep?"

Sleep is important. Obviously. Has anyone ever told you why? Well, your pituitary gland secretes growth hormone during sleep, stimulating tissue generation, organ maintenance, muscle building, fat breakdown, blood sugar balance, and free radical repair. Sleep is basically an antioxidant for the brain.

If you have trouble sleeping, you don't need me to tell you that your body is stressed. You know it. You *feel* it. The imbalanced hormones. Imbalanced blood sugar. They tell you loud and clear something is wrong.

When I work with clients one-on-one, we review their diurnal patterns. That's a fancy way to describe a person's typical twenty-four-hour routine. When do you wake up? When do you go to bed? What stresses you out in between? If you're my client, I'm your detective. I want to know how you feel throughout the day. I look at your schedule in chunks. Where are your cortisol surges throughout the day? I can see what your pattern is, then adjust your macronutrients during meal times to fit with your life, your job,

---

[10] https://www.framinghamheartstudy.org/.
[11] "Most Heart Attack Patients' Cholesterol Levels Did Not Indicate Cardiac Risk," Science Daily, January 13, 2009, https://www.sciencedaily.com/releases/2009/01/090112130653.htm.

your commute, whatever. You know what to eat and when so you don't crash and burn. Every recommendation is different because everyone's life is different.

What I can tell you, the person with trouble sleeping, is you probably need more vitamin B$_5$. This nutrient "shuts down" the neurotransmitters that keep you alert throughout the day. When a client tells me, "I can't shut my brain off," I reach for the B$_5$.

I also recommend regular exercise, progressive relaxation, and balanced blood sugar. You already know about exercise and relaxation. Physical activity is best in the morning or early evening, not right before bedtime. Even twenty minutes of jogging on the treadmill can improve your sleep. As for progressive relaxation, you're teaching yourself the difference between tension and relaxation in your body. You concentrate on your body—starting with feet, moving to your head—and focus on complete and utter relaxation of each part. Once you get used to this, you may fall asleep before you reach your head.

If these tips don't help, you need to balance your blood sugar. Nighttime blood sugars are often too low, which wakes you up. Getting your daytime blood sugars in check will help the nighttime levels to balance out. Forget how to do this? Refer back to the Rock Bottom Thyroid Reset, eat right again, and enjoy your sleep. Sweet dreams!

"Which exercises support my thyroid?"

You know you're supposed to exercise. Our bodies are designed to move. We're not supposed to be a tree. By this point in the book, you know I favor moderate aerobics, cardio, and light activities that get you moving, such as yoga and walks outside. What else? Add resistance training with weights to the list (more on this below). If you have a gym membership, you have at your disposal every option to slim down and get strong, from circuit training to free weights to belly dancing class.

If you have a thyroid problem, the wrong equipment or routine can make your condition worse. Listen to your body. If you're reacting to weight gain by pushing yourself harder, longer, and faster, you'll hit a wall—and gain more. Weight loss takes so much energy, and you have none to spare. Your thyroid is shot. Your adrenals are shot. Blood sugar, shot. Until you repair these, your body is not letting go. Heal yourself first. Then worry about weight. I once overheard another thyroid patient say, "I don't care how tired I am. I don't care if my hair's falling out. I just don't want to be fat." You don't have to be her.

Back in the day, a Billy Blanks workout system called Tae Bo came on the scene. I bought the five-DVD set and went to town. I followed his exercise calendar like a job. I also ate low calorie. I couldn't wait to see the pounds melt off. So I did two or three workouts at once. We're talking up to three hours in one session. Guess what? I didn't lose weight. I did lose my energy. Many years later, I did the same thing with spin classes. High intensity. I hung in there. I was proud of myself! Still didn't lose weight. I had epic endurance, though. If I'd tried to run a 5K race, I bet I could've made it.

Have you ever seen that person at the gym who sprints on the treadmill or hangs onto the elliptical for dear life? That's working too hard. Not effective at all. For people with thyroid problems, terrible. You're better off slowing your pace and intensity. Again, let your body be your trainer. It's okay to challenge yourself. After all, great strides happen outside the comfort zone. Slight modifications to workout intensity, treadmill incline, and weight resistance challenge you, but not to that dangerous "white knuckle" point. That's not even fun.

Speaking of not fun, nobody likes the guy who lifts weights, grunts so everyone notices, and drops them on the floor after two repetitions. *We get it—you want the gains.* For people with thyroid issues, muscle-mass maintenance is important. Getting ripped is not. Modest weights are as effective at building muscle as heavy anyway. The right weight for you is pretty hard to lift for the last few reps of the exercise. If it's super easy to whip off twenty bicep curls, that's too light. When you choose the right weight, after some trial and error, you will feel "the burn" (lactic acid) afterward, but not like you can't move for three days. When you push your muscles to the limit, they break down and repair, a process that causes some soreness. That's normal. Just don't get to the point of pain and injury. No one gets a medal for lifting a bunch of weight . . . unless it's a competition, I guess.

Being smart about your workout isn't only about what *not* to do, it's what you should do. Do you feel good about yourself when you do abdominal workouts like sit-ups or crunches? Probably. But you also need to make sure your entire core gets a workout. That includes the entire area below your chest down to your hips. Welcome to your stabilizing muscles. One hard, big movement like sit-ups doesn't help them. Same goes for your stabilizing muscles everywhere else, such as those in your joints. You need stability everywhere to protect you from injury. The back, hip, shoulder, and ankle muscles often get neglected. There is a reason why ACL knee reconstruction rehab, for example, focuses on tiny muscular contractions to stabilize that knee for future activity. These exercises seem pointless. The movements are miniscule. But they work.

My point to all this? When you exercise, exercise for function. I practice functional nutrition *and* functional exercises. You may not be exercising to compete, but you should exercise to function day to day and stay healthy and injury-free. Notice what I did not say—weight loss. We all know that an exercise routine can reduce body fat, strengthen your heart, and build healthy muscles. The question is *how.* The answer is cardio, resistance, and flexibility.

Cardiovascular exercise is any activity that increases your heart rate. That means *any* activity that affects your heart rate. Running, cycling, walking the dog, whatever. What matters are frequency, intensity, and time. If playing tennis with your kid or mowing your yard gets your heart rate up, that's cardio.

Training with weights (or body resistance) is essential. Lean muscles improve your health. Research shows that lifting weights lowers your chances of metabolic syndrome.[12] Metabolic syndrome is a cluster of risk factors, including waist-to-hip ratio, blood pressure, and blood glucose. Fall into metabolic syndrome and you're at higher risk for heart attacks, strokes, and diabetes. Resistance training also improves ligament and tendon strength, which improves your stability. Weightlifting can help you maintain a healthy weight because lean muscle tissue is metabolically active (i.e., fat burning). Resistance training, according to the Centers for Disease Control and Prevention (CDC), can raise metabolism as much as 15 percent![13] To reap strength-training rewards, train each major muscle group (arms, legs,

---

[12] "Lifting Weights Protects Against Metabolic Syndrome, Study Suggests," Science Daily, October 23, 2012,
https://www.sciencedaily.com/releases/2012/10/121023124404.htm.
[13] Rebecca A. Seguin et al., "Growing Stronger: Strength Training for Older, Adults," Centers for Disease Control and Prevention and Tufts University, https://www.cdc.gov/physicalactivity/downloads/growing_stronger.pdf.

etc.) two to three times per week. Give yourself a day or two of recovery in between. You don't need a gym membership or bulky equipment at home to resistance-train. You can use body weight, dumbbells, exercise machines, bands, cords, or an old tire in your garage for that matter! Like cardio, you can strength-train anytime, anywhere.

Flexibility is also important for reducing energy and improving overall performance in our day-to-day life. Everything from tying our shoes to lifting heavy boxes. Cardio and resistance training can tighten our ligaments, tendons, and muscles without proper stretching. We just don't function as well. Flexibility decreases as we age anyway. At minimum, perform at least one stretch that targets each major muscle group—chest, back, quads, hamstrings. Warm up for at least five minutes so your muscles aren't "cold" going in. If you find stretching boring, try a formal exercise that not only stretches the body but improves strength and balance as well. Yoga is ideal. Hold each stretch for thirty seconds. Repeat. Stretch to tightness, even slight discomfort. Don't stretch to the point of pain.

For anyone with a thyroid condition, the goal is to find efficient exercise that combines strength training with cardio. This is key. By adjusting weight and repetitions and paying attention to heart rate, you can make vast improvements in your health and body composition. Follow this protocol: resistance training twice per week, cardio twice per week. And be sure to stretch!

"How should I eat on holidays and vacations?"

Eating well is a human journey. Humans make mistakes. That's okay. Self-care means not beating yourself up over the gluten brownie you ate. Nobody belongs on the all-or-nothing train. Besides, when you make choices that make you feel better, it's easier to abstain from foods that drive your body crazy. Well, most of the time. Not always during holidays, on vacations, or at parties. Food becomes the focus of these events, but you can plan ahead, make the most of it, and enjoy yourself.

First of all, eat a balanced whole-food breakfast. For example, eat eggs cooked in coconut oil along with some sautéed bell peppers and onion. Or have a quality protein smoothie. Get full in the morning, and it's easy to eat well all day long.

After the eggs or smoothie, go for a walk. I know this is hard if you're hosting a gathering, preparing the food, or both. Get up even fifteen minutes early and get active to set the tone for the day. Maybe even add a walk after dinner with family or friends to break up the day so you're not lounging around and eating. You'll feel *much* better.

Whether you're cooking or not, stick to the basics. Rich comfort foods are tradition on most holidays. Either make or offer to bring something you want to eat, like protein and veggies. Then save the goodies for after the meal. If you want to have candy or other sweets, just plan to be off plan. Whatever that looks like for you, decide what you *really* want. Then have it. Don't feel guilty. And don't worry that you've lost all progress on your nutrition goals. Just enjoy it without overdoing it (one piece of pie is plenty) and move on.

Keep yourself hydrated all day. Headaches are common when you're dehydrated or eat high-sodium foods, which is common on holidays. Balance it all out with good hydration. Good nutrition can come later. You'd be surprised how much fun you can have on your next vacation or the next holiday with extra water, a nutritious dish, a walk, quality breakfast, and a little mercy.

"I have a food addiction. HELP!"

Have you ever wondered why you struggle with the sugar and caffeine you get from quick-fix, on-the-go foods? Do you have trouble with *not* being able to stop eating? Do you have to "clean your plate" because you feel guilty about starving kids in . . . wherever? The explanation is something called the bliss point, which I'll explain in a moment.

But first, I want you to know you're not alone. More than half of American adults are overweight, with forty million people obese. This, of course, goes right along with the increase of prescriptions for blood pressure, cholesterol, depression, anxiety, and more. Children are at risk as well because high-carb "frankenfoods" are more available and are promoted as "kid friendly." Advertisers target our children, and we fall for it! Poor diets over time rival other nasty habits like tobacco. Yes, really.

This can set us up to fall into a vicious cycle of trying to control our calories, feeling like crap, then going back to those addictive processed foods! Well, it's not your fault. These foods are manufactured to get you stuck in this cycle. Ever heard these slogans before?

"I'm lovin' it."

"It gives you wings!"

"Bet you can't eat just one."

Herein lies the problem. Most of us *can't* eat just one. And I'm not just talking about the potato chips that made that last phrase popular back in the 1980s. There is actual science behind foods that keep us hooked.

Now, I'm not saying you have zero responsibility. You have a choice to inform yourself and put the foods in your body that will benefit you and not work *against* you. Now, on to the science. Have you ever bitten into something and thought you'd just found heaven? Welcome to the bliss point. Food manufacturers add simple sugars to foods you wouldn't think are sweet so you'll keep coming back. The food industry's goal is to create craving. Nothing does it better than sugar. Ever looked at the ingredient label on a bottle of ketchup? Go look. You might be surprised . . . and disgusted. Did you know that Yoplait yogurt has twice the sugar of Lucky Charms cereal? That's crazy! Yogurt is supposed to be a "healthy" snack. Fat-free foods are so popular that these companies replace fat with sugar, artificial sweeteners, or both.

Another guiding principle to cause addiction is sensory-specific satiety. When we eat food with big, overwhelming flavor, our brain sends a signal to our body to quit eating. But junk food like Coke and Doritos were specifically designed to be not quite overwhelming to the senses. That way, the brain doesn't tell us to stop eating. In fact, it says, "Keep drinking! Keep eating!"

I could go on with different examples of well-known products that are made to keep us eating like it's a job. Everything from flavored sodas to Lunchables to Prego spaghetti sauce has cost millions of dollars to research and develop. This investment, of course, resulted in billions of dollars in sales. Food is business, after all.

My point is to get you thinking differently. To understand that your addiction or draw to processed foods is not your fault. Now that you know different, you can do different. You can get a handle on your processed junk food habits by flipping back to the Rock Bottom Thyroid Reset any time. Not everyone cares what's in their food. They just want something easy to prepare that tastes good. Stay away from sugary drinks long enough and you start to thirst for water. Not Coke. Not fruit juice. Water. That's only possible when you treat your body as you deserve to be treated. The Rock Bottom Thyroid Reset helps you do just that.

"What do I do about family, friends, and gatherings of people who don't care?"

I recently went to a social gathering. There was not one thing I could eat. Not one. Not even salad. I sat there and drank water. I didn't care. It wasn't a big deal. I got something to eat later when we left town. No big deal. No drama.

When you change the way you eat, not everyone changes with you. In fact, those closest to you may try to sabotage you. Like family. Sometimes they suck. They assume you're trying to get attention. They make it awkward. Instead of preparing dairy-free, gluten-free food your thyroid lets you eat, they serve you buttered dinner rolls and get offended when you don't touch them. *My food isn't good enough for you? What's wrong with you?* Yep, you're the weird one for driving four hours to visit family but caring enough about your health not to eat with them. Their attitude reflects their guilt that they should be eating differently, too, but aren't. That's a whole other story.

In any case, expect to find yourself in a similar situation. More than once. I sure have. So when you do, stand up for yourself. Your knowledge about what supports your body and what doesn't empowers you. You know what you need, and you don't have to hope and pray someone else prepares it for you. If I'd been hungry at the family gathering, I would've left to buy my own dinner. Usually I prepare a dish I know at least one person will eat. Do the same, and you'll avoid a lot of grudges!

"Should I intermittent fast?"

We've all heard of religious fasting. Did you know fasting can improve your health? Specifically, fasting decreases inflammation, improves your insulin sensitivity, balances blood sugar, uses your own fat as fuel, improves brain function, boosts human growth hormone, improves cellular repair, maintains muscle mass, improves cholesterol and triglyceride levels, supports your immune system, and extends your lifespan. Another fasting benefit is simplicity. You don't have to plan your life around meals. Once you get into a rhythm, you can just eat to satiety. But that's not the final reason to give fasting a try. What about the reason you bought this book—your thyroid?

Done properly and gradually, fasting benefits anyone with a thyroid disorder. Fasting supports production of T4 and T3 as well as conversion of T4 into T3, the thyroid hormone that makes you feel energized and focused. The only concern with fasting is caloric intake. Too few calories for too long of a time, stresses your thyroid. It won't produce the enzymes your body needs. As long as you eat nutrient-dense meals and get adequate minerals such as selenium, iodine, zinc, and vitamins A and D, you'll be fine.

In the basic fast, you eat your meals during a twelve-hour window. For example, you eat dinner at 7:00 p.m., then eat breakfast after 7:00 a.m. You're giving your digestion about four hours to work. Then your liver has another eight hours to do its thing.

A new brand of fasting has come along called intermittent fasting (IF). Despite the elaborate name, IF is just an extension of basic fasting. This twenty-four-hour cycle allows an eight-hour eating window. Eat dinner by 7:00 p.m., then breakfast after 11:00 a.m.

Fasting is open to variations and experimentation. Try it and see what works for you! If you're that person who doesn't eat breakfast,

IF is ideal for you. Eat only between 11:00 a.m. and 4:00 p.m. It's okay to use IF a couple of times a week. Or, after your body has adapted, you can fast daily. Quick word of caution: if you're on medications that require food, adjust your fasts accordingly. Okay, I lied—another word of warning is disordered eating. People who struggle with emotional eating can fast for the wrong reasons. *One meal a day! I'm going to start there!* That's not good. Fasting is a system; it's not about "perfect" eating. No such thing exists.

You might be wondering what, if anything, you can consume during your fasting period. Easy—drink pure water as often as possible. Black coffee, tea, and unsweetened sparkling water are acceptable. For some, the caffeine in coffee and tea may raise blood sugar, then insulin. You can buy a cheap blood glucose checker and strips at your local pharmacy if you want to learn how you respond to these or any other beverages. If anything triggers your blood sugar and insulin, don't drink it during your fast. That's why you should avoid anything with artificial sweeteners during your fasting window. Believe it or not, these can cause a blood sugar rise and insulin surge. It's like our bodies get tricked into digesting anything sweet as if it's the real thing, whether authentic sugar or artificial.

Some people modify their fast with a "dirty fast" during their window. This means you might drink some calories to help your body adjust to long periods without food. Think coffee with almond creamer, bone broth, or a green smoothie. These don't affect blood sugar and insulin like a meal does. But if fasting doesn't bring you results, keep your fasts clean rather than cutting calories during your eating window.

"Why are my female hormones jacked up?"

No hormone is separate from another. When one hormonal system (like your thyroid) gets shunted, the other hormones take up the burden and work harder. For example, birth control messes with a woman's thyroid numbers.

That's why I always talk to my female clients about their cycle, their fertility, and their future. Thyroid disorders may prevent ovulation, the release of an egg for fertilization.[14] Women with hypothyroidism have an increased risk for ovarian cysts. In severe cases, women produce breast milk even when they're not pregnant or breastfeeding! During actual pregnancy, imbalanced thyroid hormones can harm the fetus and cause thyroid problems in the mother after birth, such as postpartum thyroiditis. That's not the worst of it. Thyroid hormone deficiency can cause severe morning sickness, miscarriages, preterm delivery, stillbirth, and postpartum hemorrhage. This same deficiency can cause early onset menopause (before forty or early forties).

The good news in all this is that the impact works the other way, too. Improve your thyroid health and you improve every other system in your body, from your ovaries to your adrenals.

---

[14] "Thyroid Disorders in Women," Johns Hopkins Medicine, https://www.hopkinsmedicine.org/health/conditions-and-diseases/thyroid-disorders-in-women.

R

CHAPTER 8

Up, Down, Forward, Together: My Personal Invitation to Meet Others Who Get It

"Tiffany has been invaluable to me. She spent time with me and customized a diet and nutritional supplements plan for my needs. Tiffany is full of knowledge and experience, some of it personal, as she has several issues herself, making her an excellent wellness nutritionist. If she suggests a plan, you know she has researched all options. I have complete trust in her. Tiffany has helped me where others could not. I have received so much help and education from her, I feel confident making many nutrition and supplement decisions myself. I still call her for help with specific issues, and she remains a great source of help."

— Glenda J., Duluth, Minnesota

I know it's hard.

I know how hard it is to start over—*again.* How hard it can be to put into practice new habits to improve your health. Especially if they go against what mainstream medicine has told you.

Especially if you have a career, a family, or both. But you know what? You *can.*

You can do these things. You can change how you feel. You get the ball rolling. You gain momentum. You feel better. You're motivated to keep going, to keep improving your health on your own terms. You don't have to take the path your doctor laid out for you if it's not working. I remember how broken and devastated I felt when I thought I had no choice. When I heard my doctors telling me, "This is how this works. This is how you're going to feel now. It's just your new normal. You just need to deal with it."

You don't have to feel that way. You do have a choice. It's your choice to feel better. You don't have to be a passenger on your road to sustainable good health. "Well, they put me on this prescription because they didn't want me to gain any more weight. I felt horrible on it, and then I gained even more weight." That's life in the passenger seat. Instead, you can be the driver of your own well-being.

Several years ago, I had a client who was overweight and suffered from brain fog. She was the go-to person for everything in her home and at work. There were a lot of inescapable external stresses in her life. With an eighty-hour-a-week job and a family member suffering from a terminal illness, she needed all the brainpower she could get.

This client completed my one-on-one program that extends the Rock Bottom Thyroid Reset to twelve weeks. Not only did she lose forty pounds, her husband lost forty pounds too just by eating dinner with her. Nothing else. Not all meals. *Just dinner.* Her brain fog also cleared up, making it easier to handle the stress in her life. Along with boosted mental and emotional stamina, her blood sugar, sleep, food sensitivities, gut health, skin, and energy all improved. She went from depressed to glowing. She was a joy to be around.

A year after this transformation, deaths in the family took their toll on her. My client went off track, gained weight again, and got burned out. She didn't stay that way. I'd given her the tools to take care of herself. She cycled through the reset again, underwent vitamin and mineral testing with me, and corrected what had gone wrong. Within a couple of weeks of restarting the reset protocol, her brain fog dissipated and her energy returned.

Why am I telling you this story? Because it's real life. It's not a fairy tale complete with a happily ever after. In real life, life goes on. After we lose the weight, get the sleep, accomplish the health goal, life happens. Ups, then downs. Like my client, you can still choose to move forward—even if you find yourself slipping back to your rock bottom. If you need some help, let's talk. Here's how.

The Thyroid Breakthrough Session: Your Step-by-Step Plan for What's Next

When it comes to your health, how do you navigate the winding journey ahead called life? When you veer off the path, what do you do to get your health back as soon as possible? How do you optimize your next time through the reset for your specific situation? Like most things in this book and in life, the answers are different for everybody.

I'm inviting you to make this personal. Not on your own—I'm offering you a chance to get personalized feedback. What support do you need on your journey right now? What does it look like? What are your hidden nutritional deficiencies? What advanced issues could you be struggling with that you hadn't thought of before you read this book? Is there a food you're struggling to reintroduce? Whatever is keeping you from becoming the next thyroid patient success story, we can face it together.

If you're ready to get the personalized help you need to achieve sustainable health, reach out to me and let's schedule your free thirty-minute Thyroid Breakthrough Session today. No high pressure to "buy now." I'll simply give you the facts—what I do, how I can help, and what you can do for now. Your free session is just as much for me as it is for you to determine if we're a good fit to work together or if I can help by referring you to a different holistic practitioner. Either way, you'll come away with options and a plan to get you in the right direction. That's not all. During our Thyroid Breakthrough Session, you'll also get:

● My feedback on what's next for you in your thyroid journey

● The confidence to speak up for yourself

● Questions to ask your doctor

● Vindication—no, you're really not crazy!

● Specific symptom remedies suited to your situation

● Tangible hope that you *can* feel better

● Realistic expectations about your progress

● The truth about the underlying cause of unexplained symptoms

● Quick tips you can try right now to feel better without a huge financial burden

How can we possibly cover all of this in half an hour? Here's an example. Let's say you come to me with concerns about your blood sugar. We'll talk about how to heal your gut, how to manage the stress in your life, and which foods will help. I'll recommend you download my free seven-day meal plan to balance your blood sugar using food alone. Oh, you have histamine intolerance and can't eat avocado? I'll email you my recent newsletter about which enzyme you probably lack, one that helps break down histamines. As a result, you'll relieve some of your symptoms by the end of the week so you can tolerate more food.

All this in only thirty minutes, and it's free. Compare thirty minutes of answers to years of unanswered questions. Clients often tell me, "I wish I had a disease so at least I knew what it was and how to deal with it." Is that you, too? If so, it's time to stop wishing and start acting. You know what they say—you can pay for your health now, or you can pay for sickness later. The Thyroid Breakthrough Session is only an investment of time. What do you have to lose?

Weight?

Stress?

Depression?

Put down this book right now, and go schedule your free thirty-minute Thyroid Breakthrough Session at

www.rockbottomwellness.com/breakthrough.

Nutrition for Thyroid Health: A Safe Place for People Like You

Like me, you've probably had to walk your thyroid health journey alone. I formed a community so we (and others like us) never have to again. Nutrition for Thyroid Health is a free private Facebook group where you can ask your thyroid questions and get answers from me and from others on this journey.

Imagine surrounding yourself with literally hundreds of people who have symptoms similar to yours. They get it. They know how hopeless life seems when the doctor says, "You're fine. Just eat more carbs and take this prescription." They know how frustrating it is when family and friends pick a restaurant where you can't eat anything—and they don't even care. Say goodbye to feeling alone. When you join my free group, you can expect to find:

● A tight-knit group who are all in this together

● Weekly live Q&A sessions with me

● Fun seasonal recipes you won't find on Google

● Other members' techniques to boost your thyroid

● New research from mainstream and alternative sources

● Useful infographics and guides to make this stuff stick

- Vitamin and supplement deals up to 20 percent off retail price
- Real stories from real people that give you real hope
- Encouragement on your hard days, praise on your good ones
- Money-saving bulk shopping tips for easy snacks and meal plans

If you want to join a community that feels like family, just go to www.rockbottomwellness.com/group. Introduce yourself and ask the question that stumped your doctor. It's free, and it's worth it.

A Few Words Before We Meet Again

Most health books I've read end with a chapter that basically says, *Well, that's all, folks! Hope you enjoyed reading. That's everything you need to know for the rest of your life. Bye forever.* Then three pages of eye-roll-worthy acknowledgments that wrap up the book.

Rock Bottom Thyroid Treatment isn't most health books. This is no one-and-done motivational pick-me-up. Come back to this book anytime you like and bookmark, dog-ear, and highlight like crazy. Need a quick dinner recipe? Bookmark. Need a refresher on the best source for omega-3s? Bookmark. Binged on your grandma's Thanksgiving cooking and need to repeat the Detox Phase? You guessed it—bookmark.

I also want to part with the conventional self-worship that closes most books. That's not me. This book told my story, a story among millions. You probably saw yourself in seasons of my life. Perhaps in my clients' as well. You're coming away from this book empowered, educated, and excited to take back control from a medical establishment that profits off long-term misery. I want you prospering as you live a rich life of health, wholeness, and happiness.

So, is it time to say goodbye? Nope. Just . . .

Until we meet again.

R

Glossary

Antithyroglobulin antibodies

Antithyroglobulin antibodies are produced against thyroglobulin, a thyroid protein. The presence of these antibodies indicates that an autoimmune process is happening—your immune system is attacking your thyroid gland.

Free T3

T3 is the active form of thyroid hormones. Free indicates that the hormones are unbound, meaning they are available to your body.

Free T4

T4 is the inactive form of thyroid hormones. Your thyroid converts T4 into T3.

Hashimoto's disease

Hashimoto's disease is an autoimmune thyroid disease indicated by elevated levels of thyroid antibodies. Hashimoto's is the most common cause of hypothyroidism, but it is possible to fluctuate between hypo- and hyperthyroidism.

Hyperthyroidism

Hyperthyroidism is overactivity of the thyroid indicated by low levels of thyroid-stimulating hormone (TSH).

Hypothyroidism

Hypothyroidism is the condition of a low-functioning thyroid indicated by high levels of TSH.

Reverse T3

When the body is under constant stress, the thyroid converts T4 thyroid hormones into reverse T3 rather than free T3, meaning the T3 hormones are not available to the body and therefore do not support normal thyroid function. Individuals with elevated reverse T3 may have normal numbers for other markers, but high reverse T3 levels indicate that normal hormone conversion is not happening, which is a cause for concern and usually indicative of chronic stress.

Thyroglobulin

Thyroglobulin is a thyroid protein used as a tumor marker. This protein is of major importance for making T4 and T3.

Thyroid cancer

Thyroid cancer is indicated usually by a nodule on the thyroid gland. Thyroid cancer can spread to the lymph nodes. There are four types of thyroid cancer. From most treatable to most severe, the four types are papillary, follicular, medullary, and anaplastic.

Thyroid peroxidase (TPO) antibodies

Like antithyroglobulin, TPO antibodies are used as a marker for autoimmune thyroid disease. It is elevated when the immune system is attacking the thyroid.

Thyroid-stimulating hormone (TSH)

Thyroid-stimulating hormone is a negative-feedback mechanism. Basically, TSH levels tell you how well the pituitary gland is talking to the thyroid to regulate how much thyroid hormone is produced.

Thyroidectomy

A thyroidectomy is the surgical removal of all or part of the thyroid gland usually performed to treat thyroid cancer, a goiter, or some other severe thyroid condition.

R

Acknowledgements

I'm so grateful to the many people who helped make this book a reality.

To Steve Flaten, my husband and greatest support. You have always encouraged me to do what I need to do.

To my sweet girls, Allison and Oliva, for your unconditional love and understanding during some crazy times.

To Mom, Shireen Grinager, who has always been there to listen and offer love and support that only a mother can.

To my late father, Jon Grinager. I know you're always here. I always remember "Life is Good'" because of you.

To my sister, Staci Kost, for always cheering me on as one of my biggest fans.

To my intelligent, hilarious, supportive, and loving friends, the Fab Five: Robin Salander, Kelli Odden, Kathy Klath, and Stephanie Hammes. You've taught me the importance of lifelong friendships and have shown me there is no better feeling than laughing until it hurts. Thank you for always having my back and supporting me on my journey.

And to the nutritionist who began my healing journey and to all the patients I get to help because of that first appointment. You all encourage me to keep moving forward and help those who desire to thrive, not just survive.

Printed in the USA
CPSIA information can be obtained
at www.ICGtesting.com
LVHW052349151023
761173LV00009B/426